SHUT UP AND RUCK

THE ULTIMATE SOFA-TO-SELECTION PERFORMANCE GUIDE AND JOURNAL FOR ASPIRING OPERATORS

TF VOODOO

ISBN: 979-8-9881260-1-0

❀ Created with Vellum

We build good Green Berets from good Soldiers.
We build good Soldiers from good citizens.
We build good citizens from good men.
Learn to be a good man.

I learned to be a good man from the most honorable man I know.

This book is dedicated to him.

Thanks Dad.

TABLE OF CONTENTS

INTRODUCTION

I know of no better life purpose than to attempt the great and impossible. - Nietzsche

Day 1, or One Day.

Before we jump right in, I thought it might be helpful to apply a little context for this book. If you are reading this, then there is a fair chance that you got here via *Ruck Up or Shut Up: The Comprehensive Guide to Special Forces Assessment and Selection*. Welcome back. If you read *RUSU* then you might understand just how upside-down SFAS can be. If you didn't read it, then stop now. Go read it and come back. I will use RUSU as a basis for many of my recommendations and I won't spend much time rehashing the literature or explaining precisely why you need to be *stronger than the fastest runner, and faster than the strongest lifter*. If you're headed to SFAS then you are headed for deep water. RUSU tells you just how deep that water is, this book will show you how to swim, so to speak. In this book, we move past establishing my bona fides and we jump right into getting shit done.

If your goal is to successfully complete Special Forces Assessment and Selection (SFAS), then you are in the right place. Today is *Day 1*.

Time to get to work. If you're just *kicking the tires* of your next thing or wandering through the marketplace of fitness ideas, then this is perhaps a *One Day* thing. Maybe you're not headed to SFAS and you're simply looking for your next fitness challenge. You're curious. There is nothing wrong with that. You like the struggle, and for some reason, you seek hardship. You crave an intense fit lifestyle, and you enjoy the results. You don't have to be headed to the Sandhills of Camp Mackall to be fit. Keep reading and see if this program sounds right for you. You don't have to be waiting for The Sandman to ambush you in order to feel compelled to work hard. But what better place to be than on the path to elite military fitness? The sort of fitness that our Nation's most capable special operators require. That's what this book is truly designed for.

This book is essentially two parts. The first nine chapters of this book are the explanation part of this process, the science so to speak, for the performance journal. The second part, the performance journal, is where the rubber meets the road. You don't have to read any of the first nine chapters of explanation. If you're just looking for a workout regimen that will prepare you for the rigors of SFAS then you can simply skip this part and go right to work. But some folks enjoy a little explanation. As such, we cite no small amount of literature, but this isn't necessarily a full literature review. We want to give you some information and show you some resources if you want to do some more independent research, but primarily we want to get to the meat of the matter.

The journal itself is that meat, *The Program.* Day by day, lift by lift, and step by step. You can find other perfectly fine journals on the market, but most are essentially just blank books; there is no programming. You are free to (or, worryingly, left to) find your own program. But you might run the risk of your journal not accommodating the specifics of your program. Not so here. In *Shut Up and Ruck* the journal *is* the program. In this journal you are prescribed exactly what to do every single day. I (we actually, you'll meet the team soon) will tell you what exercises to do, the number of reps, what mileage and pace, and what to do for building mobility, assembling skills, and engaging in deliberate recovery. We even give you a reading list (finally, IYKYK), mental prep exercises, and guided mindfulness sessions. We go so far as to tell you how to sleep. We are taking out every excuse that we can. So you can read the first nine chapters to get deeply related to the knowledge behind the program, or you could jump right in and start executing. Choose your own adventure.

250 Hard

You have likely heard of *75 Hard*, the transformative mental toughness program promoted by Andy Frisella. It's a simple concept with often revolutionary results and that is exactly why it enjoys so much popularity across such a broad cross-section of enthusiasts. It is excellent, but it is challenge for challenge's sake. *Shut Up and Ruck* is different. This is *250 Hard*. This is challenge for Selection's sake, the ultimate goal. Eight months of specifically programmed prep across physical, cognitive, and interpersonal domains with a specific SFAS focus. No alterations, no compromise, no excuses. Work your ass off, do the program, and you will put yourself in a position to be measured against the highest standards in the harshest environment you could imagine. SFAS is different, so this program reflects that reality.

There are a few terms and phrases that I will use repeatedly, almost nauseatingly so, in this manuscript. This is not from lack of creativity or difficulty with language, vulgar or otherwise. I suffer from neither of these fucking maladies as anyone who has sat with me for a cocktail can attest. I am a world-class storyteller and a native-speaking shit-talker. Rather, I will use these terms and phrases repeatedly because they are important. I want you to focus on them. They deserve to be committed to memory. You will also find that these repeated mantras will often seem simplistic. Sometimes overly so, and this is also deliberate. *Simple, not easy.* That's one of those phrases. Remember it.

This book is a bit of a coup in the fitness environment. It is anti-marketing. Our advertising budget is zero dollars. The team of experts that have guided me have received no compensation. There are no subscriptions. You buy the book once, you own the whole program, and the rest is entirely up to you. The fitness industry (and make no mistake that it is indeed an industry) is one of the most competitive and crowded spaces to navigate. It can also be incredibly lucrative. Americans spend around $800 billion (depending on your source) every year on their never-ending quest for washboard abs, barrel chested pecs, and chiseled physiques. A quick look around at your fellow Americans reveals how elusive this can be. So this industry finds itself in the desirable position of being both the fox and the lion (see Machiavelli). To this end, the fitness space remains clouded in hype, misinformation, proprietary formulas, and no small amount of snake oil. Lots of guarantees, quick fixes, and scams. Take this pill or rub this cream or eat this seed. That stuff doesn't work and there are no free lunches in nature.

The disheartening thing about this environment is that if you just want accurate, reliable, and valid fitness advice you must navigate through all of the bullshit to find it. And the really disheartening thing about this environment is that the answers are shockingly simple. *Simple, not easy.* There are no secret formulas and there is no real mystery to solve. If you want to lose weight, then you have to burn more calories than you consume. If you want to get stronger, then you have to progressively overload your muscles. And if you want to build up your cardio base, then you have to put in the time slowly increasing your aerobic threshold. [1] So this book and this program is anti-marketing. No secrets. No hacks. No proprietary formula. We have posted our "secret formula" all over social media. Here it is, you may acknowledge this as exceedingly simple and a bit of *no-duh.*

---

1. Yes, I know that this is a touch unsophisticated and that there is some nuance to these topics. There are medical conditions, genetic markers, certain medications and such that complicate these equations for some. But when I see a fat person cite their glandular issue, I often wonder just how many beer-battered glands they ate...if you catch my meaning.

The Formula

- Lift Weights- 3 days a week - Bench, Squats, Deadlift, Row, Shrugs, Overhead Press.
- Run- 3 days a week - 90 minutes per session in Zone 2 without stopping.
- Eat clean.
- Stop drinking booze.
- Rest and sleep like your life depends on it.

That's it. That's the formula. But that's just generalized fitness. The sort of fitness that might see you live a long and relatively healthy life. The sort of generalized fitness that keeps you out of a nursing home should you slip and fall in your advanced years. The sort of fitness that keeps you from an endless bevy of "life-sustaining" pharmaceuticals. Normal stuff. In this case, we are talking about Operational Fitness. The sort of fitness that *Operators* need, not to put too fine a point on it. And this sort of fitness can be clouded in even more mystery. Not so normal stuff. You have to contend with Obstacle Courses and Rucking. So, we will add to the Formula:

- Rucking- Field based progressive load carriage, usually 2-3 times a week, focused on short intense sessions.

You must prepare for building and carrying insanely heavy apparatus. The Combat Fitness Test (formerly known as the Combat Readiness Assessment) is waiting for you. There is relentless and continuous high demand work...day after day after day. This is the kind of stuff that you need to be successful at SFAS. Abnormal fitness. This is the "secret." The hack. The proprietary formula, if you will. Not the work, but the environment in which that work must be performed. If you do not understand SFAS then you cannot program for SFAS prep. You can understand generalized fitness, but SFAS is just different.

I won't spend any time critiquing other programs other than to say that I find them lacking, particularly in ruck programming. Since we have well-established in RUSU just how important rucking is for SFAS success, the fact that other programs get this critical component so miserably wrong is grounds enough for dismissal. There are great coaches, decent programs, and lots of good intentions. But I don't think that they offer a complete package, and you can't afford to go to SFAS on a half-assed plan. Choose your experts wisely. Choose your programs like your success at SFAS depends on it.

The Team

I chose my experts wisely in preparing this program. There is so much information that went into building this that I would have been overwhelmed without expert counsel. I had no shortage of very smart folks that wanted to collaborate, and I had to be a bit miserly in sharing my time. So the folks that I am presenting here are the cream of the crop. As awareness of our efforts grows, we will introduce many other team members. We want to build a network of like-minded trainers, coaches, and performance specialists that can be available to you. We are not gatekeepers; we are tour guides on your path to elite fitness.

I chose four experts across multiple domains – endurance, performance nutrition, cognitive performance, strength, mobility, injury prevention, and skills development to name a few. One of the things that you will note is that this operational fitness stuff is very cross-functional. It's impossible to be an endurance expert and not have a good understanding of mental resilience. It's improbable to be a strength specialist and not understand mobility and flexibility. And it is intolerable to be an athletic performance specialist and not understand the interconnectedness of performance nutrition. So, while I may sophomorically list them as singular domain experts, they are cross-functional, multi-domain experts by nature. This is one of the reasons why I chose them to coach me and why I want them to coach you too.

I label Mr. Dave Hsu as my endurance coach, but he is so much more. First, he is a retired Green Beret officer, and we all know that retired Green Beret officers are as elite as they come. Dave commanded the Special Forces Underwater Operations School (SFUWO) at Key West. The cornerstone of SFUWO is the Combat Diver Qualification Course (CDQC) which has a hard-earned reputation as being the most physically demanding course in the Army. I am biased, but the best ODAs are Combat Dive Teams, and the best Green Berets are Combat Divers. Dave spent his career at the tip of the operational fitness spear. When Dave retired, he started a second career in Counter Threat Finance positions at Combatant Commands and at the Pentagon in the Office of the Under Secretary of Defense for Intelligence & Security. He has been coaching triathletes, marathoners, and cyclists professionally since 2010. He is currently the head run coach for the Naval Special Warfare Preparation Course in Coronado, CA which prepares SEAL and Special Warfare Combatant Craftsman Candidates for their respective selections. Yes, the SEALs need the expertise of a Green Beret to prepare for the rigors of the maritime environment. It is what it is. Coach Dave has his B.S. in Exercise Science, he is a National Strength and Conditioning Association Certified Strength and Conditioning Specialist, an American College of Sports Medicine Certified Exercise Physiologist, a USA Track & Field Certified Coach, a USA Triathlon Certified Coach, and Road Runners Club of America Certified Coach Level 2.

Coach Dave is a certified and credentialed expert, but he is also a practitioner. He understands this endurance stuff like no other because he lives it every day. I like to think of myself as a rucking *enthusiast*, but Dave is an endurance *freak*. As I write this, the last two times that I talked to Dave he was in the midst of punishing himself. Once, he was just finishing up a full distance triathlon. He wasn't coaching it; he was running it himself. Which he won. This is something that he does regularly. He's retired and he chooses to do this stuff. The other time I talked to him he was in the middle of the Pacific Ocean...swimming between the Hawaiian Islands...for fun.

"Hey Dave, how are you doing?"

"Good, I'm just swimming."

"Oh, cool. Glad that I caught you poolside then."

"Oh no, I'm on a boat."

"...So, I guess that you're doing an open water swim today?"

"Yeah, were doing a relay swim between the Islands..."

"...umm, like, off the California coast?"

"...WHOA! We just had another whale breach the surface right next to us!"

" ...A WHALE....wait, ANOTHER whale!?! Where are you?"

"...We're doing a relay between the Hawaiian Islands and I'm taking my rest on the support boat. We have a pod of whales that's been keeping us company all night," he said way too casually.

I thought to myself, "I don't think they're keeping you company, brother. I think they're *hunting* you. When you enter the water, you enter the food chain." But what I said was, "Well, good luck then. Send me a note when you get feet dry." He was swimming in the ocean, at night, with the dangerous marine fauna. FOR FUN! So when you see the endurance progression and the exquisitely planned runs, that's Dave pushing you. The guy that runs full distance triathlons in his "retirement" and swims with whales. You had better keep up, because he isn't slowing down. And neither is SFAS.

I categorize Dr. Sean Burkhardt as my mobility guy, but that is doing his expertise a real disservice. Dr. Burkhardt holds Board Certifications in Sports Chiropractic, Physiotherapy, and Functional

Neurology, with a special focus on brain health, injury rehabilitation, and concussion management. He is also a certified Functional Medicine Practitioner and a triple-certified NSCA Strength and Conditioning Coach. He is a certified Strength and Conditioning Specialist (CSCS), a certified Tactical Strength and Conditioning Coach (TSAC-F), and a certified Special Populations Specialist (CSPS). He is a National Academy of Sports Medicine certified Corrective Exercise Specialist (CES) and certified Performance Enhancement Specialist (PES). Sean is also Functional Movement Systems certified for Functional Movement Screen (FMS), certified Selective Functional Movement Assessment (SFMA), certified Fundamental Capacity Screen (FCS), certified Screening and Assessing Breathing: A Multidimensional Approach (FBS), and certified Y-Balance Testing (YBT/MCS). If it seems like I'm trying to overwhelm you with credentials, it's because I am. Dr. Burkhardt isn't some CrossFit Level 1 weekend warrior. He's a board-certified expert who has been trained and qualified to within an inch of his life, so I trust him implicitly.

Beyond all that *plebian* physical stuff, Sean could really be best described as a *Neuro-Performance* expert. This is where his skill really shines. In Chapter 7 you will see his work most clearly. It is academically dense material and there is a good chance you will get 'contact asthma' from all of the nerdiness, but his grasp of the complex connection between your brain and your physical performance is amazing. By the way, Sean is already researching and writing on the cognition of Close Quarters Battle. He has taken the same attention to detail that he applied to the ARSOF Attributes in Chapter 7 and applied it to CQB. If you're a tactical athlete or shooter, you just found your new best friend. Listen to what he says about the Attributes to get started and get a spot in his virtual locker room for his CQB cognition insights. You'd better get on his dance card quickly because he is about to lead a whole new trend in maximizing shooter performance.

Dr. Burkhardt runs Boulder F.I.T. Health and Performance along with his wife, Halley. Halley is a biologist with a Master of Science in Nutrition and Human Performance. She also is a Certified Functional

Medicine Practitioner. Her clinical work at Boulder F.I.T. gives her a unique understanding of performance nutrition that perfectly synchronizes with my approach to SFAS prep. No show, all go. She is exceedingly practical and her expertise cuts right through all of the typical nonsense I often associate with the 'diet industry.' You aren't on a diet; you are fueling for performance. Every time I read some nonsense quasi-science loon chirping online about the next food trend, I hear Halley reminding me that we already know what works and what doesn't. Our job is to get you to execute the plan, not craft some bespoke dysfunctional menu and supplement atrocity. Basics build champions.

Finally, we are lucky enough to have Mr. Nate Toft join the team. Nate has spent the last 10+ years learning and understanding the factors that facilitate peak performance. He completed his graduate work from Miami University, with a concentration in Performance Psychology. He has had the opportunity to work alongside individuals from all walks of life and with a variety of performance contexts (high level executives, amateur and professional athletics, and tactical populations). Nate is a Cognitive Performance Specialist and a Master Resilience Trainer with the US Special Operations Command. Most importantly for us, Nate spent half a decade at the US Army John F. Kennedy Special Warfare Center and School. That's right, Nate worked at SWCS where he trained directly with SF Candidates and SFAS Cadre. He understands the Selection environment uniquely, because he coached the Cadre on what to look for and he coached the candidates on what to show them. He has walked Team Week and seen the cognition and resiliency in action. Literally an expert on cognitive performance at SFAS. His expertise and insights are amazing, and he is a skilled teacher. You are going to learn from the best.

So *Shut Up and Ruck*, guided by these experts, occupies a unique position. This little niche between generalized fitness, bullshit fitness, and abnormal fitness is where this book finds its real value. In the following pages we will take the very simple (not easy) principles of diet and exercise, sleep and recovery, and human performance and human nature and apply to them my unique understanding of SFAS. Some of the protocols that we will follow are not fully endorsed by the credentialed protectorate of the industry. I have no interest in preserving that environment. I am not a fitness, physiology, or psychology expert, but I am an expert. I am an expert in research design. I have taught graduate level research methodology for over a decade. I can whip up a research question, a thesis statement, or a null hypothesis on the fly. I can develop an analytical framework, craft a literature review, and artfully record conclusions and recommendations in short order. Any reasonably smart person can be trained to do this fairly easily, and I have a team of true experts advising me. The research is published, all that you have to do is read it. As such, I have evaluated the evidence and nothing that I recommend herein is even remotely controversial. I am, most decidedly, an expert in SFAS. All that this book will do is take these well-established concepts and apply them in the context of SFAS.

But this context is absolutely going to kick your ass. Ruck up...

1

FOUNDATIONS OF OPERATIONAL FITNESS

Strong minds suffer without complaining; weak minds complain without suffering. - Lettie Cowman

I nterconnected. In a word, operational fitness is interconnected. *Stronger than the fastest runner and faster than the strongest lifter.* Really strong, but not meathead strong where you can't reach your hand into the middle of your back. So flexible, too. Strong and flexible. And really fast. But not so fast that you can't bear the burden of a heavy load. So, fast and strong and flexible, but also athletic. Athletic enough that you can maintain stability across multiple simultaneous planes, you can move enormous loads, and you can nimbly move your body across obstacles. Like the Nasty Nick. Broadly speaking it's about being able to do work, do that work quickly, and then recover quickly so that you can do that work again. Your mental resiliency and cognition are huge components to this as well. We will spend significant effort in subsequent chapters applying a structure towards this specific prep effort. So each part of operational fitness gains efficacy from working with its adjacent part. The whole is greater than the sum of the parts.

Operational fitness is defined in six broad categories (we will call them pillars): strength, endurance, mobility, skills, cognition, and finally, rucking. While rucking is a hybrid of the strength and endurance pillars (and a little bit of skill, cognition, and technique), it demands its own category by virtue of its weighted importance to SFAS and its unique demands. There is just something special about the inimitable misery that rucking provides, so we must prepare accordingly. *Every important decision that you make at SFAS you will make with a ruck on your back.* Keeping these six pillars in mind, we will endeavor to address each pillar in a deliberate and meaningful way. By this, I mean that we will absolutely focus on becoming faster than the strongest lifter and stronger than the fastest runner, but we won't forget about rope climbing. I've seen more than one physically impressive specimen fail the Nasty Nick because they couldn't manage to mantle over the top of a rope climb obstacle. We also recognize that most skills training sessions are likely less physically demanding than an intense strength training session. As such, we can use skill building sessions as active recovery or even rest periods. We will also be very deliberate in that we will not do any 'vanity' exercises. No bicep curls, anterior serratus, or oblique targeting, and no made-up exercises...except for the 5x5. Trust me, it's made up but it's worth it. You'll get plenty of arm work doing chin-ups, pullups, pushups, and rows. Your core will be strong from squats, deadlifts, and overhead presses. Leave made up exercises to *the industry*. You're going to Selection, so you need consistent and disciplined execution of the essentials. All of them. Basics build champions.

We also recognize that none of us enjoy the privilege of unlimited resources. With a personal chef, a valet, a private gym and trainer, a masseuse, a physical therapist, and the funding for unlimited nutritional supplementation, damn near anyone can get really fit. I feel like Superman when I get a new pair of running socks, so I can't even imagine what a personal staff would do for me. For the rest of us non-superheroes, the most precious resource might be time. We all have lives to live. We balance many competing priorities, and we must meet many challenging obligations. So we don't have the luxury of two-a-day gym sessions, or endless physio trials, or any of the trappings of the 4-hour work week. To this end, we have carefully developed this program to remove all of the extraneous stuff and gain as many efficiencies as possible. The 5x5 Man Maker is a perfect embodiment of this philosophy. Maximum impact, minimum time, perfectly scheduled. So we will only choose the *best* exercises, the *best* methods, and the *best* protocols. We only have so many resources, so we want to stay focused. To be certain, there are many ways to skin the cat. We will use the best way for SFAS prep. When you get to the *How To Use This Journal* chapter you see just how efficient this process can be. It is as intense as you could hope for, but the law of diminishing returns is ever present. Let's break down each pillar.

Pillar 1 – Strength

We will define strength as the ability to exert physical force. Within the specific context of SFAS in that the exertion is done under extreme conditions that most athletes never contend with. It is a brutal environment. Perhaps in the parlance of exercise science, time under tension. You will be training in a gym, but you will be tested in the Land of the Longleaf Pine. There are no sets and reps at Camp Mackall. You work until you win. There is no deloading week. You are loaded until The Sandman is secure. There is no hypertrophy, or intermittence, or anabolic effectors. You go as fast and as hard as you can until the Cadre announce, "Congratulations, you've been selected." So we will be ever mindful of the totality of the exercise science, and we will endeavor to stay well within the established *best* practices. But we might allow that upside-down world context to shape how we apply that science. Some of the most well-established exercise science concepts are the concepts of periodization, specificity, progressive overload, and adaptation. These concepts will be the foundation of our programming process. We will select exercises that are as analogous to SFAS as possible. We will focus on these exercises and gradually increase the weight, frequency, or number of repetitions. We will account for the body's physiological response to training after repeated exposure and the program regularly recalibrates your loads. This is all well-established and practical exercise science, with proven exercise components, and done with disciplined regularity. Simple, not easy.

Pillar 2 - Endurance

This component of the six pillars gives us the other half to our stronger than the fastest runner and faster than the strongest lifter paradigm. We spent considerable effort in RUSU documenting the performance benchmarks for speed: 6 to 7-minute mile runs and 12 to 13-minute mile rucks for pretty much unlimited distances. But endurance isn't just about running and rucking quickly. It also becomes about recovery. Yes, you can go fast. But can you do it with that same intensity tomorrow? How about later tonight? How about in ten minutes? You don't have the training schedule for SFAS, so you simply won't know. So we need to train for that, the unknown and unknowable variable. To be truly prepped then we need to address aerobic capacity as broadly as possible, so we'll talk about this capacity as the body's ability to transport and utilize oxygen. We can also measure this efficiency with which the body can transport oxygen in the blood to the heart where it is distributed to the muscles, and the capacity of the muscles to use the oxygen received. On call horsepower with maximum fuel efficiency. A challenge under perfect conditions. A requirement for SFAS.

Pillar 3 - Mobility

We divide mobility into three broad categories to include injury prevention, flexibility and agility drills, and pre-workout sequences.

Injury prevention is further defined in terms of both preventing injuries in the broader program by building prerequisite baseline strength, flexibility, and resiliency proficiencies before vigorous strength and conditioning phases of training and in best practices and proper coaching through activities that present higher likelihood of injury. Part of this is the flexibility and agility drills. The best way to build flexibility is likely static stretching. But you can enhance that flexibility by building spatial awareness and body control through agility drills. Things like plyometric and explosive drills, balance and poise exercises, and fluidity movements. The early phases of this program will recruit these components heavily. We do this deliberately to build both self-awareness and establish strong foundations so that you can make maximal time and effort in the later phases. You can't do the 5x5 effectively if you can't squat, have poor run form, and are awkward in your ruck shuffle. So we'll build that athleticism with purpose and intent.

Pillar 4 - Skills

An under-appreciated component of operational fitness is the myriad of skills one should master. Obvious instances like rope climbing, balance (again), and monkey bars directly translate to the Nasty Nick obstacle course. But so does stuff like mantling (climbing over the rope climb anchor point), body control (weaving your body under and over obstacles), and equilibrium (balance, but at height and under duress...like at the top of obstacle). I have seen countless candidates that were fast and strong but couldn't negotiate basic obstacles. What good is being faster than the strongest lifter and stronger than the fastest runner if you can't get past the *Weaver* or the *Tough One?*

But the skills go beyond the Nasty Nick. What about manipulating an apparatus during team week? Weaving yourself, with a ruck on, around other candidates and the burdensome load, in order to rotate positions? What about climbing over a downed tree in the depths of a thickly vegetated draw, all while avoiding the wettest parts of the swamp during Land Nav? What happens if someone drops an apparatus, and you don't have the prowess to leap out of the way? I've seen more than one candidate leave Camp Mackall in an ambulance because he couldn't save himself from injury. Can you tie knots? What about tying them under pressure? You might be surprised how many teams miss a time hack because they can't disassemble the apparatus quickly enough. Fine motor skills with the weight of the world on your shoulders. So we'll build these skills deliberately.

Pillar 5 - Cognition

You can't be dumb. This is true in life and critically true at SFAS. Often described as PhDs that can win a bar fight, Green Berets are critical and creative thinkers without peer. The old axiom of 'think outside the box' simply doesn't apply because as a Green Beret you will often have no box at all. So you have to be smart. This book, and much of the narrative surrounding the SFAS prep environment, is physical fitness focused and rightfully so. But nearly all programs *only* focus on the physical fitness realm. This is a colossal mistake. What it shows is a real lack of understanding of SFAS. Novices believe that SFAS is just about the physical. Lift this, carry that, and don't quit. The truth is that the physical stuff is just the beginning. Lift this, carry that, don't quit, and resolve complex social interactions inside of a deviously manipulated environment while Cadre continually press you for explanations and elucidations. You will have 300 plus pounds on your back and simultaneously be asked to engage meaningfully in complex cognitive functions. In other words, you will be in a bar fight while defending your PhD dissertation. So if you aren't training to engage your brain whilst you "fire your posterior chain," then you aren't training properly. Maybe we should add *smarter than the fittest athlete and fitter than the smartest erudite* to our *stronger than the fastest runner and faster than the strongest lifter* mantra.

You might be starting to understand how complicated this prep stuff is. All the rules really do matter, all the time.

Pillar 6 - Rucking

Rucking performance is the number one predictor of success at SFAS; up to six times more predictive than the next metric. Every important decision that you make at SFAS, you will make with a ruck on your back. You will spend up to twenty hours or more a day under a ruck. Ruck this, ruck that. Ruck here, ruck there. Rucking, Rucking, RUCKING. RUCKING IS KING! To make matters more complicated, rucking seems to hold some secret mysticism for most people. We will present, defend, and conclude the best rucking methodology in the next chapter, but we should pre-emphasize some points here. In order to maximize your rucking performance, you must establish optimum conditions as a pre-requisite, maintain good form and discipline while training, and carefully monitor and record the multiple variables that impact that performance.

We are threading the *simple vs easy* needle very carefully here, so you don't need to record your boot/sock/insole combo on every single movement. But if you get a nasty blister that precludes you from training for a week or more, then your progress will suffer. You don't have to build bench press and squat strength before you throw on The Tick. But if you can't build that pre-requisite strength then you won't be able to stabilize that ruck on your back and that flopping load will prevent you from optimizing your performance. You don't have to train to engage cognitively while under load. You can just pop in your ear buds and distract yourself from the misery every time you go on a shuffle. But then you won't be ready for those moments at SFAS when the Cadre are assessing you and your chances of getting selected depend on your ability to think well and communicate effectively while getting crushed become suboptimal.

These are the 6 Pillars of Operational Fitness. *Stronger than the fastest runner and faster than the strongest lifter. Smarter than the fittest athlete and fitter than the smartest erudite.* This *Shut Up and Ruck* program will cover all 6 Pillars and then some. There is a lot of stuff to cover. We are just through the Introduction and Foundations, and we are already at 6,000 words. Now, if we're this deep just at the foundation, imagine how much stuff you have to address during execution! Yes, there is a lot. Let's get started.

NO SHIT, THERE I WAS...ONE THOUSAND, TWO THOUSAND...

S FAS is a great microcosm of some of the best people that America has to offer. Hard-charging, incredibly fit, humble, God-fearing, warrior elite. And some fucking weirdos. It's a bit of a numbers game, so you often get a cross-section of whatever the Army has to offer. Of course some of that offering is less suited to the SF lifestyle. When you see these weirdos in action, it can leave you scratching your head in bewilderment.

We had a guy who was a Drill Sergeant and he showed up to Selection fresh from "the trail," that is directly from Drill Sergeant duty. Drill Sergeants, as one might guess, can be real cock-of-the-walk guys. When you spend your days around powerless, know-nothing recruits, it can go to your head a bit. This guy thought that he was a real gift to the Regiment. What makes it so much better is that once you show up to SFAS, normal Drill and Ceremony stuff goes right out the window. It would infuriate him that nobody would listen to his admonishments of our non-traditional "turn that way and walk" commands.

This guy spoke exactly like you might expect, acted exactly like you might expect, and dressed the part too. In this case that meant

Jump Boots. Jump Boots, you see, allow for a pristine shine, and in Basic Training Land, this is what is important. Jump Boots do not, however, perform well for road marching. But Drill Sergeant was determined to prove himself superior, no matter what. He proudly bragged, "You young pups don't know what the 'Old Army" was like!" We recognized his false bravado.

"Hey Drill Sergeant, do you do a lot of rucking at Basic?"

"Hell, yeah. We smoke them privates!"

"I heard that you guys just have pillows in your rucks."

"Fuck that. I'll smoke you guys too! You'll see what that *Airborne Shuffle* looks like as I fly right past you!"

So the class forms up for one of the forced ruck marches and there he is, in all of his glory, wearing Jump Boots. Most guys spent months prepping their boots to wear like a slipper and perform like sneakers. But Drill Sergeant? He had other ideas. We set off on a nice long ruck and he is slowly dropping back in the pack until eventually he just fades off into the background. We finished up and most guys had completed recovery and hygiene and we noticed that he wasn't back yet.

About an hour later he comes limping into the barracks, sullen and dejected, tosses down his ruck and plops down. He is in obvious distress and it's clear that his pronounced limping is the source of his angst. We know what's going on, he knows what's going on, and he knows that we know what's going on. He slowly and delicately pries his feet from the boots and delicately peels his socks off. His feet are a bloody and mangled mess. He tips his boots over and literally pours blood from the boots. He is done. Pride cometh before the fall.

We felt so bad for him that we actually helped him carry his bags to the Camouflage Hut (the much-maligned Quonset hut for dropouts, now replaced by Tent City). But we didn't feel so bad that we wouldn't mockingly call out, "One Thousand, Two Thousand, Three Thousand, Four Thousand!" every time we saw him after that. This cadence is well known to anyone who is Airborne qualified. Whenever an Airborne Instructor calls out, "Jumpers, hit it!," you had to pop up into a strong exit position and loudly reply, "One Thousand, Two Thousand, Three Thousand, Four Thousand." It seemed fitting for the Jump Boots. Airborne Shuffle indeed.

PREPARE YOUR GEAR APPROPRIATELY. And don't be a fucking weirdo.

CHAPTER 1.5

"FIELD BASED PROGRESSIVE LOAD CARRIAGE, USUALLY 2-3 TIMES A WEEK, FOCUSED ON SHORT INTENSE SESSIONS."

The best way to build rucking performance is *field based progressive load carriage, usually 2-3 times a week, focused on short intense sessions.* This statement is at the core of our ruck programming, and it garners more criticism than almost anything else. This shouldn't be contentious, but it is. It throws the established conventional wisdom on its head. It counters decades of "that's what I did" institutional and personal momentum. Thirty years ago, the program was 8 weeks of rucks with a 6-miler week one and a 24-miler in week eight, adding a few miles each week. You started at 35 pounds and slowly moved up to 75 pounds by the final week. You complemented this with the classic body-building split of chest and tri, back and bi, and shoulders and legs. Throw in some Fartleks (remember those?) and maybe an "advanced" technique like a swim or two and there was your SFAS prep plan. For many, this remains "the plan" today. You might throw in some updates like AMRAP, or HIIT, or track repeats, but the rucking remains nearly identical. Just look at the official SWCS produced SFAS Prep plan or any of the official THOR3 plans. Some of these don't even have weightlifting! But they definitely get the rucking part wrong as well.

Most Soldiers hate rucking. It is almost seen as punishment and there is little wonder why. Most units don't train for rucking. They simply host an annual or semi-annual 12-mile ruck march event for unit validation. It becomes, predictably, an emotionally significant event. Because nobody in the unit has adequately prepared for it, there is always a marked increase in associated injury rates. Put plainly, it sucks. It spawns the 'rucking is bad for you, wear dress socks to prevent blisters, and load up on creatine and energy drinks' narrative that prevails almost uncontested. Boomer Fudd-lore bullshit. This is the reality that so much of the literature addresses. We're not unsympathetic to the misery, we simply maintain that those people aren't preparing correctly. And our recommendation is hard work, so it's bound to be unpopular. It is a relentless and intense process (just like SFAS). So lots of people predictably resist it. We should note that our training statement is not our opinion; it is what the evidence, the peer reviewed, real world recorded evidence shows us. You can certainly make an argument that "peer-reviewed" doesn't hold the credibility that it once did. But it is still the gold-standard. We should recognize that experience does matter, so your observations and practice can certainly inform your argument. But not at the exclusion of what the empirical evidence demonstrates. In the Taxonomy of Information, data and evidence outweigh narrative and anecdotes. Let's take a look at the counter-argument.

What our position doesn't say might be a more revealing place to start. We don't say the *only* way, we say the *best*. There are many ways to train rucking. You could program the antithesis method: treadmill based, set pace and weight, once every 2 weeks, focused on long slow distance. You would certainly see some sort of stimulus, particularly in poorly trained athletes. But not better than our method. Not the *best*. There is also a significant distinction to be made with how we define best. Best for what? Injury prevention or VO2 Max? Muscular endurance or flexibility? There are near unlimited variables and the literature seems to favor injury prevention. Fair enough, but we're training to get selected, not to primarily avoid injury. We define best as increased speed and weight carrying capacity. Finally, we say *build* rucking performance, not *maintain* performance. We are assuming that the athlete is beginning from a relatively low performance benchmark. Once you build to a high-performance benchmark there is little evidence to suggest that more than once a week is indicated. But were specifying the *best* way to *build*. Words matter.

The *field based progressive load carriage* component is very well established in the literature. You would struggle to find a study that concludes anything but this. *A Systematic Review of the Effects of Physical Training on Load Carriage Performance* (Knapik, Harman, Steelman, & Graham, 2012) is a fairly comprehensive meta-analysis of this component and should provide more than enough support for this conclusion to even the most doubtful skeptic. Many critics also cite that this article concludes only one weekly progressive load carriage session, not our recommended 2-3. But this isn't the conclusion in the studies that it reviews. The full conclusion is "...field-based training conducted at least three times per week that incorporates a wide variety of training modes and includes one weekly progressive load carriage." Three times a week is much more relevant, and one might conclude *at least* one weekly progressive load carriage. The conclusion is not clear in this literature, so we should continue to seek clarification elsewhere, as we have done.

The Army itself has published some guidance via the Uniformed Services University Human Performance Resources Initiative and recommends "limiting ruck marches to one every 10–14 days, planned in coordination with resistance training and cardio days." (Uniformed Services University, 2023) They base this recommendation on Technical Information Paper No. 12-054-054-0616 (Army Public Health Center, 2016). But the TIP itself concludes that this methodology:

> "...**may** provide optimal performance with the **least risk of injury**. Because exceeding four marches a month **may** unnecessarily **increase risk**, training regimens should not exceed one distance march a week. Unit mission, baseline fitness levels, other physical activities and training, as well as terrain and climate must also be considered."

Again, the focus of these recommendations is *injury prevention*, not performance. And even this recommendation includes uncertainty (may) and the caveat that mission and baseline fitness levels must also be considered. Our mission is building elite rucking performance. Our mission is SFAS. We are certainly mindful of injury prevention, but it is not the primary consideration. All of the literature that recommends rucking frequency less recurrently than at least once a week are prioritizing injury prevention, not performance gains. We also prioritize establishing high baseline fitness levels before rucking in earnest. Our methodology includes eight weeks of preparatory fitness work to include strength, flexibility, mobility, and cardio baseline before rucking is prescribed. This is exactly in accordance with the literature already cited (Orr, Pope, Johnston, & Coyle, 2010). Evidence.

We should also note the actual recommendation in the TIP is "... field-based training conducted at least 3 times per week." Why the distinction between load carriage and other field-based activities? Other than injury prevention in low-fitness trainees, what is the difference in load carriage training versus any other physical training modality? There is no evidence that in a properly conditioned athlete that more frequency correlates to higher injury rates. Would any reasonable credentialed coach program any other physical event only 2 or 3 times a month? What sort of performance gains could one realistically expect training an activity every 10-14 days? One should be mindful of overtraining, but what about undertraining? Can you realistically expect optimum performance gains with such infrequent training? Which method is better, twice a month or twice a week? Not what methods are acceptable, rather what is the *best*.

Finally for frequency, we absolutely must layer on top of this the analysis of the specific training mission of SFAS. No reasonable person believes that training twice a month would be adequate to build rucking performance for Selection. There is no evidence to support such a conclusion. At SFAS you will be rucking nearly every day for the duration. During Gate Week you will have several timed rucks of an unknown distance. If you are fast enough, you get to go to

Land Nav Week. Here you will be rucking every single day. You will
be under a ruck for 8-10 hours a day. Again, if you're fast enough and
you can manage the inherent cognitive load and find your points, you
earn a shot at Team Week. In Team Week you will be under a ruck,
and then some (see: The Sandman) for upwards of 22 or 23 hours a
day. And finally, the Long-Range Movement: seemingly endless miles
on a bruised and battered body with likely shredded and compromised feet. Twice a month prep? Good fucking luck. In the Knapik, et
al meta-analysis the training frequency is as varied as 3-5 times a
week, while the intensity and duration were manipulated (Knapik,
Harman, Steelman, & Graham, 2012). So following well established
exercise protocols we can conclude that 2-3 times a week is the *best*
frequency for building performance, particularly SFAS level
performance.

The final variable in our recommendation is intensity. You can
manipulate intensity with three common variables: speed, distance,
and weight. Some studies cite duration, but duration is a derivative of
speed and distance. We use all three of these variables in our
programming with our benchmark variable being speed. And
because we focus on *short intense sessions,* we can focus our programming manipulation on the speed and weight. We develop our understanding of short intense sessions from five key studies, Soldier Load
Carriage: Historical, Physiological, Biomechanical, and Medical
Aspects (Knapik, Reynolds, & Harman, 2004), Optimizing Operational Physical Fitness (NATO's Research & Technology Organization, 2009), The Development of a Preselection Physical Fitness
Training Program for Canadian Special Operations Regiment Applicants (Carlson & Jaenen, 2012), The Role of Strength and Power in
High Intensity Military Relevant Tasks (Maladouangdock, 2014), and
Optimizing the Physical Training of Military Trainees (Orr & Pope,
2015). We should also note that these studies and many of their cited
sources, further support the 2-3 times week frequency conclusion.

What these studies conclude is that intensity matters, particularly
with regards to load carriage training. Intensity must be sufficient to
elicit a physiological response proportionate to that recommended

for cardiovascular and metabolic fitness development, with the speed and weight gradually progressed to levels that meet programming needs (Kraemer, et al., 2004). These studies also note that one of the key factors in injury prevention is fatigue and that fatigue sets in at the tail ends of duration, so shorter is better (Bloch, et al., 2023). Some studies cite distances as short as 2-3 miles and even .25 mile sessions (Poel, 2016). We conclude that this is too short, except for specific targeted sessions, to achieve the fitness, technique, and misery management elements of rucking specific fitness. We determined that the 'sweet spot' of maximum intensity and sustainable misery balanced with *relative* injury prevention is 5 miles. We could have chosen 4 and we could have chosen 6 as the evidence is inconclusive at this level of detail, so we assessed 5 miles as optimum. You can certainly train for longer distances, but your intensity will suffer, and intense sessions are better. Remember, we are looking for the best method.

There it is. The thesis statement: *The best way to build rucking performance is field based progressive load carriage, usually 2-3 times a week, focused on short intense sessions.* You have the argument, the counter-argument, the logic, the evidence, and the literature review. We only cite about a dozen sources here, but there as many as several thousand articles to support these conclusions. This is an evidence-based conclusion, supported by countless peer-reviewed articles, following all of the most accepted and well-established fitness programing principles. Just because it goes against what you did, or what your buddy recommends, or what Skull and Dagger SpecOps Fitness, LLC recommends doesn't mean much in the face of the overwhelming evidence. You are free to program your rucking train-up in any manner that you choose. But if you aren't doing it as *field based progressive load carriage, usually 2-3 times a week, focused on short intense sessions* then you aren't doing it the best way. Choose your experts and your expert advice carefully. SFAS is an upside-down world and requires a deliberate and informed prep.

NO SHIT, THERE I WAS…FIELD BASED RUCKING

We continue to emphasize the importance of field-based training, or train like you fight. This is especially true for rucking. The more than you can replicate the varied gravel, hard-packed sand, and sugar-sand trails of the Pineland the better for your progress. We had a guy who could have used some additional field-based ruck training, but I'm not sure how you might replicate a scenario for this specific training.

For our final Long Range Movement, we started on the Camp Mackall compound (what is now called the Rowe Training Facility) and followed the winding trail for a few miles before coming to a long straight miles-long sandy road that made up the rest of the route. What we ended up doing was essentially a 'down and back course,' where you walked down this road for several miles to a turn-around point where waiting Cadre would record your roster number and perhaps weigh your ruck for compliance. Then you were turned around and sent back down the road where you would repeat the process at the other end. Back and forth through the night.

As you might imagine, you are incredibly fatigued at this point in the process. Your feet are in pretty bad shape. It felt like my toes were falling off. Your legs are just there, neither strong nor weak. Just there, barely holding you up. Your back and traps felt permanently welded to your ruck. It had been pressed so forcefully for so long that you simply melded into one being. And your mind was in pure survival mode. Barely coherent and drained beyond measure, your cognitive functioning is...*compromised*.

It was not uncommon to sit down and change socks or make gear adjustments during this extended movement. Some guys would sit down to do a little foot maintenance and simply fall asleep, overwhelmed by exhaustion. You had to be particularly careful that when you took a break that you didn't return to the course and continue on your way in the wrong direction, essentially negating that portion of your movement. I was so paranoid that I set my compass and was diligent about checking my azimuth even though I never left the road.

One guy, Big Gay Al, didn't use this technique. And it cost him. He ended up not only falling asleep several times, but he also got lost. Twice. When he eventually jostled himself awake, he popped up and started trotting down the trail to make up time. Except he was moving in the wrong direction. He walked up to one of the checkpoints and after the Cadre recognized how far behind he was they asked what was up. He shot back in a pained exclamation that can only be described as an over-the-top version of Scarface's Tony Montana "Say hello to my little friend" line.

"Candidate, what the fuck are you doing? Why are you so slow?"

"Sarge, I know what I'm doing! But my feet are KILLING me!"

We calculated that he ended up doing an additional 10 or 12 miles. He made it, but he paid the price for his poor technique. Big Gay Al got selected and I later served in Group with him. He was a solid NCO and a great storyteller. Whenever we got together the "*My feet are KILLING me!*" line never fails to get a good laugh.

EVERY IMPORTANT DECISION that you make at SFAS you will make with a ruck on your back. You are well-served to train like it.

2

STRENGTH PROTOCOLS: STRONGER THAN THE FASTEST RUNNER

What should each of us say to every trial we face?
This is what I've trained for, this is my discipline! - Epictetus

Nobody ever said that they wish that they were less strong; certainly no SFAS Candidate. You might be so big that you wish to be faster or leaner or more mobile, but you can never be too strong. This is especially true at SFAS, where your strength will most definitely be tested. I've recently spoken to several unsuccessful Involuntarily Withdrawn (IVW) Candidates who claimed that their SFAS out-counseling included remarks that they needed to be stronger. And more than a few who Voluntarily Withdrew (VW) and cited their perception that they were too weak and were only hurting their Team. So even though we don't have definitive strength benchmarks derived directly from Selection standards, we can surmise that you need to be strong. Likely stronger than you think.

The Six Lifts

Basics build champions, we are going to focus on a few very

fundamental lifts, and we will seek to master these compound movements to maximize our gains and concentrate our efforts into functional strength. These lifts are the Bench Press, Squats, Deadlift, Row, Shrugs, and Overhead Press. We have deliberately whittled the list down to the very basics and we have been thoughtful about our choices. You can masticate over our picks all that you'd like. You can make the argument that the Incline Dumbbell Fly induces more hypertrophy when conducted with a movement tempo of 2/0/1/0 and is directed at a .87 x 1 RM and enjoined with an eccentric vs concentric focus and is maximized with a .85 gram per kg of BW of plant based protein taken within 46 minutes of the mid-point of maximal activity, blah, blah, blah...you can make that argument. Or you could Shut Up and Ruck. The Barbell Bench Press is what we selected. It is a well-established foundational lift. It builds significant musculature in the upper body, it is an excellent predictor of overall upper-body strength, it is infinitely customizable, and it is low risk. Lay on your back and press big weights off your chest. Barbells, dumbbells, kettlebells, Bulgarian bags, lead pipes, ammo crates. Whatever you have, lay down and shove it off your chest. It's best with a stable padded bench and standardized weights, but the movement is as fundamental as it gets. So stop pressing for an argument and start pressing the weight. Once you've spent some time working the bench, or you've sustained a limiting injury, or you've plateaued with a standard form, you can start to explore the merits of incline vs. decline, fly vs. press, or barbell vs. dumbbell.

So to get us started, Bench Press it is. We should also note that we assigned a baseline bench press pre-requisite benchmark before you should start rucking. What does a bench press have to do with rucking? The bench press, in addition to building a barrel chest (if you're trying to become a *Barrell-Chested Freedom Fighter* you need a barrel chest!), helps create a strong and stable core. If you don't have a strong and stable core when you start rucking, you will struggle to stabilize the load of the ruck. The ruck will, in essence, flop around and control you. This flopping motion wastes energy and may even lead to injury. You will struggle to coach every possible efficiency out of rucking under even perfect conditions. Imperfect conditions of a flopping unstable load are simply untenable. So the bench helps your rucking performance. You will also do no small number of pushups. You need to prepare for the Physical Fitness Assessment (PFA, sometimes called the PFT or Physical Fitness Test) which includes Hand-Release Pushups (HRPU), so your chest will get plenty of attention without adding superfluous accessory lifts.

Next is the Squat, specifically the Back Squat. This is the part of the program where guys start compensating. They complain, "I don't like back squats because I hurt my neck once." Or, "I get a deeper stretch with a split squat." Or my favorite, "I get too bulky in the thighs when I squat." Shut up. The program is squats. Shut up and do squats. If you want to do some variation, then have at it. If you want to do lunges, then go right ahead. If you want to just skip squats and rely on your rucking, then you will suffer the consequences. The program is squats. Deep squats, ass to ankle, with fully open hips at the top. Control the weight on the way down and explode up from the bottom. You will be working, eventually, with very heavy weights so proper form is imperative. Squats are critical to building the appropriate musculature to properly stabilize a ruck, along with the core stability produced by the bench press. If you can't squat, then you can't ruck. At least you can't ruck at the high level that you will need to. The relationship between squats and Team Week should be obvious. The Sandman, Pails of Pain, Mulan, and others are all very similar to the top position of a back squat. In high carry events, you will almost always carry the burden across your back. A few will require you to shoulder the burden, but the stabilizing core components will call on the squat functionality. If you need to substitute a Front Squat or Overhead Squat to protect your neck, then you might reconsider your decision to go to Selection. The Sandman would like to have a word with you, and he'll be whispering in your ear whilst perched on the back of your neck. So squats are best performed as Back Squats.

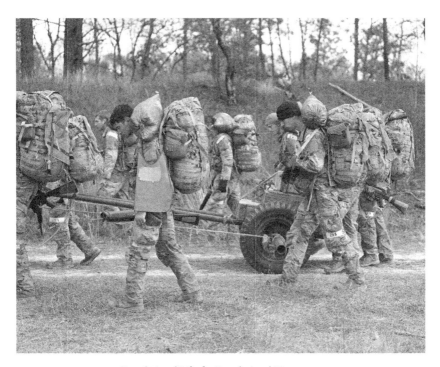

Foundational Lifts for Foundational Movements

The Deadlift is next on our list of essential lifts. The Deadlift, like the bench press and squat, is about as foundational and essential as you can get. Critics might argue that Deadlifts are counter-indicated because of the higher risk of injury. Deadlifts can, and will, include very heavy weights (culminating at twice your body weight) but there is nothing inherently dangerous about the movement when done correctly. You probably already Deadlift every day. You bend over, grab stuff, and stand up regularly. Your daily routine is likely not very heavy, but the movement itself is as functional and foundational as they come. The application to SFAS is obvious. Team week is essentially four consecutive days of hundreds, if not thousands, of dead-lifts. Every time you touch an apparatus or a pole or an ammo can, you are bending over, grabbing something (something pretty heavy in this case), and standing up. When you stop to rest and set down the load, you do a deadlift. When you stop to switch positions, you do a deadlift. When you stop for another map check, you do a deadlift. All day long. During Land Navigation week you do a deadlift every time you doff and don your ruck. The deadlift is essential to your performance at SFAS, so it is also essential to our prep.

The next foundational lift is the Row, the bent over barbell row specifically. We are less dogmatic here as there is sufficient evidence to warrant other variations. Chest supported dumbbell rows, single arm rows, T-bar rows, even seated rows on a machine will get the job done. But we advocate for the bent over barbell row. The row will work the entirety of your back, but it will also work your forearms for grip and the biceps as well. You will want a thickly muscled back to balance out your growing barrel chest. Practically speaking, well-developed trapezius muscles are required to support your ruck straps. You will thank yourself for your diligent work in the gym when you are out on the sandy trails at Camp Mackall and that ruck is really pressing on you.

We will support this development with shrugs. We prefer dumbbell shoulder shrugs, but a barbell shrug is acceptable. Shrugs primarily work the trapezius, but they are also uniquely relevant to SFAS as you will do lots of single arm carrying. Whether it is water cans, ammo crates, or telephone poles you will be low carrying repeatedly. The combination of rows, shrugs and pull-ups is not sufficient to develop the requisite grip strength so you must continuously work this modality. A set of spring-loaded grip trainers at your desk or in your car, towel (fat bar) grip pull-ups, farmers carries, and a rock-climbing finger board are all helpful. Simply put, you can't get too much grip training. You must program additional grip strength training. The question that you are asking is something like what exercises, how many different types, and how often should I do them. The answer is yes. You should do them all, all of the time, as often as you can sustain it. You are going to need more grip strength than you can imagine.

The last weightlifting exercise is the Overhead Press. The OHP will work your upper back, chest, and shoulders primarily. We want to be very deliberate with our shoulder work. The shoulder is a relatively delicate structure. The literature suggests a strong genetic predisposition for shoulder injury, so we want to exercise some caution here (Longo, et al., 2019). There is no reliable database of SFAS prep injuries, but our experience suggest that shoulders are one of the most common training injuries. We assess that improper form is the likely culprit. The prevalence of CrossFit style Metabolic Conditioning workouts with the emphasis on speed and maximum repetitions that often sacrifices form is a good example of this phenomenon and kipping pull-ups are an excellent illustration of this. At Selection, you will find yourself overhead pressing often, especially during Team Week. So the OHP is an ideal prep. However, in a world of bodyweight bench presses and double bodyweight deadlifts, the OHP is relatively much lighter.

These six lifts, along with some calisthenics, will be the basis of our strength protocols. You may note that while we are prescribing specific exercises, we are adhering to the philosophy of pushing and pulling. That is, when we work our lower body, we will push with the squat and pull with the deadlift. When we work our upper body, we will push with the bench press and pull with the rows. And when we work our shoulders and upper back, the foundation upon which we will build our monument to rucking, we will push with OHP and pull with the shrugs. The Schedule A/B format, basic exercises, and basic training philosophy. No patented procedures and no proprietary regimens. *Basics build champions.* Once we establish some baseline 1 repetition maximum strength numbers we will use an alternating training schedule, known as periodization, to optimize your strength and muscle hypertrophy. We will alternate between schedule A and B monthly wherein Schedule A will focus on 4-8 repetitions with heavier weights and 3-4 sets per exercise with 2-4 minutes rest between sets and Schedule B with 8-15 repetitions with moderate weights and 2-3 sets per exercise with ~90 seconds rest between sets. This procedure of select exercises with specifically programmed work/rest cycles allows us to maintain very high intensity without too much concern for overtraining. You will work, very hard, but for a short intense duration. You will work each lift twice in a week. Not necessarily twice in the same calendar-week, but twice in every 7-day cycle. There are two lifting workouts, and you are simply alternating them. Just follow the program. Each strength workout should only last about an hour, perhaps a touch longer if you require an extended warmup/mobility session. This means that you must be focused. Gym time is not time to socialize or check in on your social media. Get off your phone and get on the bench. The only status update you need to make is *Doing Work* and the likes and hearts you need are waiting for you on Day 21 at Camp Mackall. We will provide a targeted warmup and mobility menu in Chapter 4, and you will customize this routine based on your functional movement screening results and your progression in the program. The menu is adaptable and customizable for you, so you have some skin in the game every day.

Consistency is critical for your maximal growth.

NO SHIT, THERE I WAS... STRONGER THAN THE FASTEST RUNNER

A *War Story* to help put into perspective the insane level of strength that you need for SFAS. Just surviving a "normal" Team Week day will have you doing hundreds of repetitions of squats, deadlifts, overhead press, and farmers carries. I've seen teams move under load for 23 continuous hours, just to change socks, choke down a cold MRE, and get right back into another 23-hour day.

And that's a "normal" day. Some days it strays into the abnormal all the way to the downright absurd. As teams make their way through the day, they stay fairly close together along the routes. You'll see teams jockey for position to avoid getting stuck behind a slower team on some difficult terrain. Cadre know the routes and events well and when you see them start to congregate by the road you know something is about to happen. When you see them break out their camp stools and form little viewing parties you can be assured of a real struggle session.

There was one particular route on a little downhill leg, that got badly washed out with deep ruts and high curbs. I'm talking about a sunken trail with 5-foot-high sides and a 4-foot gully separating the wheel tracks. This sort of terrain is impassable with an apparatus. Unless you have a team of well-conditioned workhorse Candidates.

One poor team entered the gauntlet, under the watchful eye of the Cadre peanut gallery, with a particularly poorly constructed apparatus. As they were portering this wonky apparatus down the trail they had to leapfrog Candidates into each rut and gully to sort of muscle the thousand-pound monstrosity through. As the painstaking process continued, the massive weight would shift and slide, and the lashings started giving way.

I watched a team take 3 hours to move less than 30 feet. After the apparatus finally just crumbled under its own weight the Cadre initiated the infamous "Cadre Takeover." Under 'direct leadership and guidance' from a frustrated Cadre, the team had to haul the remnants, piece by piece, out of the gully, back to the top of the incline, and rebuild the apparatus entirely. After a too-long, red-light headlamp, and 'fuck this' fueled rebuild session the team had to renegotiate the perilous route. They were not allowed to take their 70-pound rucks off the entire time. They finished the day as the sun was rising.

No matter if you build the perfect apparatus, tie the best knots, or follow the ideal route you will need to be strong for SFAS. Stronger than the fastest runner and likely far stronger than you think.

YOUR DISCIPLINE in the gym is the only thing that will save you.

3

ENDURANCE PROTOCOLS: FASTER THAN THE STRONGEST LIFTER

Fatigue makes cowards of us all. – Vince Lombardi

Simply put, you are going to run a whole bunch of slow miles for a few months and do some specific strength and conditioning exercises for injury prehab and such. Simple, not easy. Then you will start rucking slowly and running some faster miles. Then you're going to put it all together and ruck and run really fast in combination. This will take months to do correctly. You must do the first part before you can do the second part. And you must do the second part before you can do the last part. It's going to be a slog. It's going to take discipline. There are no shortcuts. You aren't preparing for *Michael Scott's Dunder Mifflin Scranton Meredith Palmer Memorial Celebrity Rabies Awareness Pro-Am Fun-Run Race for the Cure*. You are preparing for SFAS, and this is the best way to do it. If you don't do the prehab stuff, then you're likely to get an injury. If you don't build your cardio base, then you won't be able to sustain a competitive pace. If you don't do the ruck and runs as a combo, then you won't benefit from the mental prep and resiliency component. We don't call the 5x5 *The Man Maker* for nothin'.

SFAS is an intentional mystery, but we do have some idea of how fast we need to be, for both rucks and runs. We outlined in *RUSU* the following:

> We know that you must be able to run 2 miles in at least 15:12 for the PFA, so 7:36 a mile. We also know that SWCS recommends a sub-40 minute 5-mile run. That is a minimum benchmark. We also know that run performance is a strong indicator of Selection success. Similarly, we know that there are some specific rucking time benchmarks (Velky, 1990). They might seem a little dated, but my experience confirms these times to be excellent benchmarks for performance. It's fair to say that faster is always better, both rucking and running. We can use these various data points to establish a logical speed benchmark: 6–7-minute mile run targets and 12-13 minute mile with 55-pound ruck targets.

Despite the requirement to report to SFAS with a valid PFA within 30 days of reporting and the generally well-published performance benchmarks, a shocking number of Candidates show up unprepared. I understand some performance jitters, but some guys look wholly out of shape. I've seen multiple guys get a 20-minute 2 miler. That's 10-minute miles. Unburdened and unladen. On the very first event of SFAS. Oof. Don't be some guys. It's especially important to be mindful of these established benchmarks because we *don't* have similar benchmarks for strength. Thus, we will be really pushing in the strength domain, and we will use these speed benchmarks to anchor our strength performance...faster/stronger. We also know that the correlation between run time and overall Selection success is quite pronounced (see chart). So, we want to be fast.

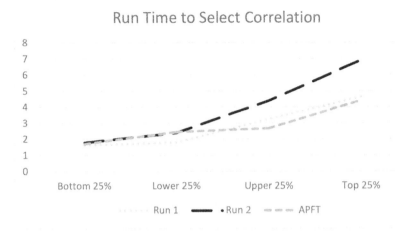

Run Time To Select Correlation (Farina, 2019)

In order to get fast, we are going to approach building your endurance in a methodical and deliberate manner. Weeks and weeks of base building, supported by specific strength training and injury prevention/pre-hab, followed by weeks of capacity building. We will build speed eventually, but not until we get strong enough to support the intense effort required and not until we build an aerobic baseline. From an endurance perspective your end state is to be able to run and ruck maintaining a specific pace, as described above. The journey to get you there is the process. We will provide you a very sound framework with specific workouts. But as you develop, you may note some lagging performance and start to question the process. So, let's talk about process for a minute.

Coach Dave Hsu was the primary engine for our endurance programming. As described in his introduction, he lives, eats, breathes, drinks, and dreams endurance. You don't saunter off on full distance Ironman competitions or 15-mile open channel swims between Hawaiian Islands (honestly who does this stuff?!?) unless you are prepared. And preparing takes discipline and process. So Dave is a process guy by nature and his guidance here is excellent. He talks about his process of "chunking." Building the sort of elite endurance that you need is going to take time, so "chunking" is an effective way to manage the monotony. If your run and ruck times are falling short and you are losing perspective, then "chunk" your process. Our very first performance benchmark is 90 minutes unbroken running at Zone 2. For many, this is a virtual light year away. So Dave likes to take these spans and break the goals into time-scheduled progressions. The framework is just that, a frame. You can adapt it as your performance merits. You can do this within the individual phases and inter-phase as well. So long as you meet the performance benchmarks, the pathway is yours to choose. A very common and effective paradigm for goal setting is using the SMART method (Specific, Measurable, Achievable, Realistic, and Time-Bound). In addition, chunk your goals into daily, weekly, monthly, and long-term (quarterly). That's right, we will tell you what to do, but you need to refine your individual preparation through diet, recovery, hydration, and sleep to optimize your performance. This is part of the process of you taking ownership of your progress. Finally, use the journal to write down your goals and document your progress. Dave gave us the example of performance progressions below; note the time it takes to drop 3 minutes:

2 Mile Test Run						
Date	Date + 2 weeks	Date + 1 Months	Date + 2 Months	Date + 3 Months	Date + 4 Months	Date + 5 Months
17:00	16:30	16:00	15:30	15:00	14:30	14:00

Performance Progressions

The Physiology of Endurance:

I think inherently we know that we can't rush this process, but we don't really know why. We don't really understand the physiological processes that have to occur in order to build endurance. I know I certainly didn't know until Coach Dave broke it down for me. I was happy and content just running. But it's helpful to understand what all of that running is doing. We need to discuss how the body adapts to build this aerobic capacity. Your performance is a great deal pre-determined by your genetics (Guth & Roth, 2013). But that's not necessarily a precondition or limiting for your performance. Your training and your willpower are also significantly impactful. In other words, don't make excuses. You can't control your genetics at any rate. Your ancestors decided your genetics long ago. We will focus on your training, since this is something that we *can* control. You get to decide on your will power. We have a whole chapter to help you build it. Mindset matters.

PERFORMANCE = GENETICS + TRAINING + WILL POWER

THINK of your personal endurance genetics as your ability to naturally withstand fatigue. Can you perform fatigued? Do you have the will power to do so? The answer is that you can train for it. Understanding fatigue can be helpful. Some guys are just natural freaks. You are not one of those guys. So you need to know these markers. Coach Dave describes the two most important physiological markers to gauge your running/rucking potential as your lactate threshold and your VO2 max. This is what we will be working on. However, at SFAS you don't get points for a high lactate threshold or a high VO2 max. What matters are your times. This is how we measure performance at Camp Mackall. A higher lactate threshold and VO2max will allow you to push harder for longer, so tracking times is appropriate and simple. Let's break these markers down.

Lactate Threshold

There are many different theories, names, origins, and definitions of the concept of "lactate threshold," and some very sophisticated ways to measure it. For SFAS purposes, we will define lactate threshold as the heart rate, pace, or power that you can maximally sustain for a one hour. How long can you go fast before fatigue over-whelms you? Once your running or rucking intensity exceeds your lactate threshold, then fatigue will start to increase at a much higher rate than while exercising at below lactate threshold. Dr. George Brooks, a metabolism expert from the University of California at Berkeley has studied lactate extensively for over 40 years with some 420 publications and over 30,000 citations. From his research we now know that lactate is the most important precursor to produce more fuel—glucose. About 30% of all glucose during exercise is derived from lactate metabolism. You are producing lactate all the time, even at rest. At rest and in low intensity aerobic exercise, your body can clear the lactate easily. The limiting factor is when your exercise intensity exceeds your ability to clear lactate. This is your lactate threshold.

Lactate is primarily cleared by slow twitch muscle fibers. So to increase your lactate clearance capacity it's important to develop your slow twitch fibers which is done in aerobic runs well below your lactate threshold. Let me say that again: *an immutable, unavoidable, mandatory step in increasing your lactate threshold (so that you can run and ruck fast for extended periods) is developing lots of slow twitch muscle fibers and the best way to do that is long, slow, boring runs.* You can't skip this step. This is the foundation. You can't just start doing speed work and expect to sustain maximal performance unless you build this foundation first. The process wins every time. You don't rise to the occasion; you default to the level of your training. This is why your training is deliberate and measured. Your training will save your ass on mile 24. That other guy who just said, "Full Send!!!," will have rhabdo. You will have your long tab. Trust the process.

In a lab, lactate threshold is measured by drawing a pin prick of blood periodically while exercising at increasing intensities. This can be done running on a treadmill, a stationary bike, or rowing ergometer. Fitness wearables, such as Garmin, can estimate this without a lab test. In the chart that follows, we look at a good recreational runner. This athlete can maintain a pace of about 10 miles per hour without exceeding their lactate threshold. Their body can manage the workload without significant fatigue. But once they go faster than 10 miles per hour you see a little spike in lactate. In other words, the level of exercise is producing more lactic acid than the body can clear. They are beginning to fatigue. This is sustainable, but not for too long. Once that athlete reaches 11 miles per hour you see a significant spike in lactic acid, to an unsustainable level. So your goal is to build the body's ability to process that lactic acid, thus increasing your lactate threshold. The more slow twitch muscle fiber you build, the longer you extend that point where your threshold impedes you.

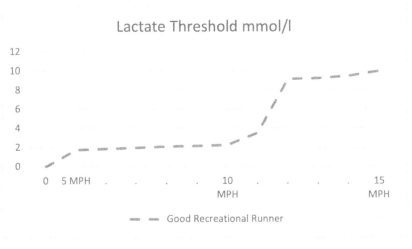

Lactate Threshold

VO2 Max

Lactate threshold is our first measure of endurance, and VO2 max is the second. VO2 max is a measurement of your cardiorespiratory fitness, or how well your body takes in and uses oxygen during exercise. It is measured in mL/kg/mil of oxygen. The average VO2 Max is about 35-40 mL/kg/mil. These numbers likely mean nothing to you, but they might be helpful as we described below. VO2 max is about 50% genetic. However, untrained athletes can increase their VO2 max as much as 95% (Laury & Tehrany, 2019). *Those* numbers should definitely mean something to you. Like with lactate threshold, fitness wearables will also measure this during your training. You might notice a little trend here: we identify a possible data point and how to measure it? If you can measure it, then you can record it. If you can record it, then you can track it. If you can track it, then you can improve it. The *mad scientist* plot thickens!

An active 25-year-old male has a typical VO2 max of around 45. The highest recorded VO2 max was 97.5 in an 18-year-old professional cyclist. The US mile record holder has a VO2 max of around 85. It's difficult to quantify what your VO2 max should be for SFAS, but you can virtually guarantee that you will catch some sort of funky upper respiratory phlegmy grossness that will make its way through the barracks. It seems that nobody escapes it, especially in the winter or wet classes, and the better your VO2 max the better you'll be able to adapt. Another way to think of VO2 max is breathing efficiency, while lactate threshold is circulatory efficiency. Critically, the relationship between VO2 max and lactate threshold is that when the VO2 max increases, so too does the lactate threshold. So they are symbiotic, but we need to train them with different modalities.

We will train to increase our VO2 max with some high intensity and interval training, but not until we establish a strong base of cardio through loads of monotonous Zone 2 running. Your speed will come, your VO2 max will come, and your intensity will come, but first we need to lay the foundation. If we don't lay this foundation correctly you won't have the performance in the higher paces that you need and you will get inconsistent (bad) data that will make tracking your progress difficult. Be patient, trust the process, and know your role.

Identifying Limiters

It's just human nature that we train what were good at. This is why you see so many guys walking around with thick backs, bulging traps, and barrel chests while teetering on toothpick legs. Show me a man with skinny legs and I'll tell you he is no man. Training legs sucks. It takes discipline. They are big muscles with massive work capacity, so you need to move huge weight, intensely in order to grow them. There is a reason why skipping legs to train chest again is a trope. It's just human nature. And it's holding you back. We are going to do the opposite. As Coach Dave says, "We have to train the stuff that nobody else wants to, because we want to do stuff that nobody else can." And we have that luxury because we know what level of performance you need to be at to be successful at SFAS. So we are going to identify all of your shortcomings, and then were going to attack them. You're no good at pull-ups? Good, we're adding another set to your warmup. You have no aerobic baseline? Good, we're adding another session every week. You can't climb ropes? Good, that's your skills workout. No metaphorical toothpicks for you.

In endurance training, your main limiting factor will simply be fatigue over time. The endurance requirements to be successful at SFAS are extraordinary. One of the primary reasons for failure at SFAS is not just a lack of strength, but a lack of maintaining that strength over long periods of time—endurance. In addition, due to the heavy loads, the ability of a Candidate's tendons and ligaments to endure day after day of heavy loads introduces one to the term—durability. This durability can only be achieved through consistent progressive stress and recovery. One of the best abilities is availability, so being able to endure the rigors and simply survive long enough to get Selected is a challenge. Fast, strong, and durable.

Physiological Adaptations Towards Endurance

As you might imagine, these sorts of physiological adaptations take some time to manifest. You can't just do a few workouts and see instant results. There are no free lunches in nature. And it's not a simple hand wave of endurance adaptations writ large. There are several adaptations that occur and at differing rates. An aerobic workout today, physiologically, will manifest itself in physiological adaptations in the body in about five to seven weeks. We are talking about complex processes like mitochondrial biogenesis, enlargement in cardiac dimension, structural adaptations in arteries, arterioles, and capillaries, and alterations in the vasodilator capacity (Hellsten & Nyberg, 2015) (MacInnis & Gibala, 2017) (Farrell & Turgeon, 2023). And these adaptations quickly go away absent of training, as demonstrated in the table below which shows the percentage change, both positive and negative, in relation to time of training and after cessation of training. So a deliberate, comprehensive, and coordinated plan is in order.

Adaptation	12-month change from baseline	24-month change form baseline	Change 6 months after cessation of
Aerobic Enzymes	100%	120%	-120%
Oxidative Potential of FT Fibers	60%	60%	-60%
Glycogen	40%	50%	-50%
Capillary Density	40%	50%	-50%
VO2 Max	40%	40%	-40%
Cross-Sectional Area of ST Fibers	20%	20%	-20%

Physiological Adaptations

Endurance Training

Just as with our strength training, we are going to approach our endurance training with basic, foundational, and traditional training principles. The general principle of progression is the most applicable to start. In order to reduce the risk of injury do not increase weekly volume of running or rucking more than 10% per week. There is good evidence to support this increased restriction to distance, time, and speed. No more than 10% increase in any domain week to week. You will be placing a tremendous burden on your system, and we want to sustain this performance to the maximum extent possible. So you can't just add a bunch of miles stacked over a few weeks and expect to remain injury free or enjoy the physiological adaptations that we need. It takes time, patience, and discipline. We are going to divide our run programming into 5 categories using Heart Rate Zones as our metric.

When you calculate your training effort with heart rates, it is all based off your maximum heart rate (MHR) and a percentage of that MHR to gauge relative effort. There are a multitude of available formulas to calculate this, but for simplicity's sake we are going to use 220 minus your age. This is called the Fox Method. The various formulas all come out to about the same target, but if you feel compelled to calculate using a different method then so be it. Just be consistent across the program. So, a 20-year-old will have a MHR of 200 (220-20 years=220 MHR), and 75 percent effort would be a heart rate of 150.

Types of Runs

- Zone 1 [50-60% MHR] - Easy Run – Easy runs are about 1/3 of our weekly volume and will serve as our active recovery runs. The goal is to increase blood flow while not inducing a training load. This increase in blood flow will increase delivery of nutrients to sore muscles more than doing nothing. The duration for recovery runs should be between 20-40 minutes at a pace less than 60% MHR.
- Zone 2 [60-70% MHR] - Foundation Pace – The foundation pace will be about 2/3rd of our weekly volume and will serve to develop cardiovascular stamina and skeletal durability. The reason why this pace is the cornerstone for all endurance running programs is because it is the ideal pace to develop endurance and durability while minimizing risk for injury.
- Zone 3 – [70-80% MHR] - Threshold Pace - The threshold pace will be less than 10% of our weekly volume and it will be in a single weekly session of no more than 30 minutes. This pace is comfortably hard, and its purpose is to improve lactate clearance.
- Zone 4 – [80-90% MHR] - Speed Work – Speed work pace is low volume (less than 5 miles or 5% of weekly volume, whichever is less) and its purpose is to maximize anaerobic power. Intensity should be at or close to VO2max and HRmax.
- Zone 5 – [90-100% MHR] - Tests – All-out effort when marking performance for the record.

NO SHIT, THERE I WAS...100 MILE PER HOUR RUCK

You'll see all sorts of bad footcare during SFAS. We covered this extensively in RUSU, but clearly not everyone can read, as you see some wild stuff. We had a kid that was particularly bad at foot care and serves as a valuable cautionary tale. Everyone gets blisters and it's a constant battle to keep your feet in a sufficiently good condition to keep training. You end up with some wacky treatment stuff.

There seems to be this enduring legend that 100 MPH tape is infallible. 100 MPH tape is the ubiquitous standard Olive Drab Green military duct tape. It got its name because, as legend has it, it was used for field expedient repairs on helicopter blades in Vietnam. It could withstand 100 MPH winds, so it was called "100 MPH tape." But the reason that it sticks so well is that it has some strong adhesive. This is good for rotor blades, but bad for feet.

This kid was pretty desperate to keep his feet together and he decided that the only way to stay in the fight was to use 100 MPH tape. There is some merit to the technique. A small piece of tape might help with friction. But the tape doesn't breathe very well, and eventually, you have to take it off. This inevitably ends up doing more damage, usually way more, than it protects against.

And this kid did himself no favors. In his desperate attempt at relief, he fashioned a sock of 100 MPH tape...directly onto his foot. So he spent the final Long Range Movement with his foot stewing inside of this super sticky and completely waterproof sock. Heat, friction, and moisture (the blister power trifecta) with no chance at letting the skin breathe. By the time he finished, he had this blood and puss-soaked OD green booty that he had to now remove.

His foot looked like it had been "degloved." Go ahead and clear your search engine history of those other feet pics and do a quick image search for deglove injuries, but don't say that I didn't warn you. He may have won the battle, but he definitely didn't win the war. And it's safe to say that a 100 MPH ruck is a bad idea.

YOUR PREP SHOULD BE intentional so that you don't find yourself getting so desperate. Take care of your feet and they will take care of you.

4

MOBILITY AND MOVEMENT PREP

First say to yourself what you would be and then do what you have to do. – Epictetus

For this program, we think of mobility and movement prep as a foundational part of both performance and injury prevention. You are about to embark on a comprehensive, lengthy, and *severe* physical regimen that is designed to prepare you for the brutal and austere conditions that you will experience at SFAS. You are going to challenge your cardiovascular endurance, your strength, and your flexibility. You will be building muscles, developing skills, and establishing neural pathways that have remained largely untaxed until now. So pain is inevitable. But injury is another story.

You need to learn the difference between being hurt and being injured. You are going to be sore (aka hurt) but that's not necessarily injury. Injury can be very preventable. Muscle soreness from an intense workout is not the same as a torn muscle. Tender feet from lots of rucking are not the same as blistered open sores. And sore joints are not the same as a torn ligament. You will undoubtedly experience being hurt, but there is much that you can do to mitigate the risks of actual injury. So this chapter will give us a guidebook for the most common injuries that candidates-in-training experience and some methods to both prevent injury and increase recovery options in the event of actual injury. We'll also discuss optimized recovery options which should be integrated into the movement prep, injury prevention, and mobility protocols.

Injury Prevention and Treatment

We are including the injury prevention block in the mobility chapter because, as you'll soon read, many of the protocols for injury prevention are the same as for mobility and the same as for move-ment prep. Interconnected, again. "The best way to treat an injury is to prevent it from ever happening and the greatest predictor of an injury is a previous injury" (Hewitt, 2017). An ounce of prevention is worth a pound of cure, as the saying goes. If you have a history of injury, then you need to be particularly focused in your prep. So much of this advice is focused on developing the resiliency required to prevent the injury from occurring (or re-occurring), especially early in the program. A key component of this is the programming itself. We will reiterate the discussion of ruck programming and high-light the principle of establishing baseline strength in the bench press and squat before beginning rucking in earnest. You can certainly start your SFAS workout prep with a long heavy ruck (like many poorly designed programs recommend), but you are far more likely to injure yourself, delay training, and induce general misery with minimal gains than you are to see any real training benefit. To this end, we will spend some time building resiliency.

You are likely familiar with the RICE injury treatment protocol. Rest, Ice, Compression, and Elevate has been the stalwart mantra for decades. Trust the Science™. The problem is that the evidence, the actual science, doesn't support this protocol (Scialoia & Swartzendru-ber, 2020). You're likely far better treating an injury with movement. But what movements and at what intensity and how much movement and, and, and? It can be a little overwhelming. This is where a guy like Dr. Burkhart can be critical. I choose my experts carefully and he just gets it. You can see all of his credentials (they are vast), but I am always struck by just talking with him. He listens. He's a fixer. He is quick with my favorite answer to difficult questions by saying, "It depends..." and then can launch into a detailed dissertation on all of the variables upon which it depends, simply tell you what his years of experience have shown him, give you a review of the relevant literature, or have you describe what your desired outcome is and before you've finished he has a detailed treatment protocol ready. Dr. Burkhardt and Coach Dave have transformed the way I think about coaching in general and even more so changed the way I think about digital coaching. In as little as one coaching or treatment session Dr. Burkhardt can save you weeks or even months of pain and delayed training. If you have a smartphone, then you have access to world-class performance experts. He helped shape this next section, but it is not a substitute for medical advice. If you prep dutifully, you may never have need of his services.

Because we aren't professional candidates, we don't have endless time available and resources to dedicate to complex injury prevention regimens, physical therapy, and hot yoga classes. We need to do a little analysis and focus our most limited resource, time, on the most likely injuries and address them as efficiently as possible. So we are picking the most common injuries and looking for opportunities to kill two birds with one stone. We will focus on 6 injuries that are the most common and most detrimental. They are:

- Plantar Fasciitis
- Runner's Knee
- Achilles Tendonitis
- Shin Splints
- Trapezius Impingement
- Lower Back Pain

Plantar Fasciitis (PF)

The Plantar Fascia is a ligament that spans the bottom of the foot from the heel to the toes and supports the arch of your foot. Plantar

Fasciitis pain often manifests in the foot or heel and can be excruciating and debilitating. The most common treatment is rest, hot/cold therapy, and even taping, bracing and custom orthotics. But we should endeavor to simply avoid it with some preemptive measures. The entire Shut Up and Ruck program is predicated on deliberate and ample timing, so a candidate in training has weeks of low mileage running (and months of zero milage rucking) to set the conditions and ease your body into the rigor.

We recommend the following exercises/routines to prevent and/or treat Plantar Fasciitis:

- Calf Work: seated with a band or towel, a standing wall lean, or on a platform for extended depth the simple calf stretch is one of the best ways to prevent PF. Calf strength work is also strongly indicated. Standing or seated calf raises will provide both a stretching mechanism and build structure to support the workload that the PF must endure.
- Toe Towel Work: We recommend 2 types of toe work. The first method is to grasp the towel in your toes from a seated position and lift your foot about 12 inches off the ground. This is sometimes called the Monkey Foot Towel Lift and is the first level. Early on you will find this simple exercise quite taxing, but as time goes on you can add light weights on top of the towel. The second method is to lay the towel out and lightly step on the end of the towel. Then flex and curl your toes to essentially draw the towel up under your foot, forming the foot into a dome. You are reaching out with your toes and scrunching the towel up. Again, adding light weights can be helpful as you advance.
- Ball Roll: Simply roll your foot on a hard ball, like a lacrosse ball, or a frozen bottle of water. Keeping in mind that there isn't an abundance of evidence for the efficacy of injury recovery with ice, it can provide temporary relief and control some localized

inflammation. But manipulating the PF with pressure can be helpful. Simply hand massaging often provides relief, but the ball helps target pressure deeper into the tissue.

- Good shoes/boots and insoles: It seems obvious, but not every foot is the same and some footgear and insoles just don't work for some feet. So spend some time going through the process of finding the right shoes and the right insoles. We exhaustively cover boot fitment in RUSU, but we don't really cover running shoes. We like a medium drop, medium cushion, slightly aggressive-sole running shoe. There is no need for a full trail shoe at SFAS, but you definitely don't want racing slicks. Stay away from the 'finger shoes,' they violate Rule 1.

Runner's Knee

Runner's Knee is an umbrella term commonly used to describe any one of several conditions including Patellofemoral Pain Syndrome and Iliotibial Band (ITB) syndrome. There's a good bit of evidence to suggest that genetics is the prime driver in predicting knee pain, but we find that poor running form is the common denominator that we can impact the most. So if you have a history of knee pain or have a concern of pending pain, you might benefit immensely from some coaching, especially early on in the program. Even filming yourself and watching your foot strike, leg angle, and knee position can be helpful. If you can get that video to an experienced coach (like Dave or Sean) they can often diagnose mechanical issues almost immediately.

We recommend the following exercises/routines to prevent and/or treat Runner's Knee:

- Proper Form – You can't fix something if you're just going to go back out in your next session and jack it up again. So work on developing proper form (including arm movement, which can influence your leg movement) first.

Get a coach if you need to but establish this critical component first.

- Strength Training – The knee is a complex structure and running/rucking can place tremendous forces on the joint. One of the best ways that you can protect your knee is to build strong legs. That musculature will provide the support, through the entire range of motion, that will give you the longevity that you need. Our programmed strength sessions are specifically designed to build that musculature. Stronger than the fastest runner...

- Programming – You need to build your intensity slowly. Again, we recommend never exceeding more than a 10% increase in any domain from week to week. You will note that we have 8 months in this program, we build every component deliberately, and you start very, very slowly. This intentionality is part of the injury prevention process. Trust the process.

- Good Shoes and Insoles – Imagine that. Interconnected, efficient, deliberate. Simple, not easy.

Achilles Tendonitis

The Achilles tendon connects your heel bone to the calf muscles at the back of the lower leg. This tendon is the largest/strongest tendon in the human anatomy and while it doesn't have a traditional fascial sheath, it does have a tendon sheath that is usually the cause of pain in Candidates, called Achilles Tenosynovitis. Absent of trauma, what normally occurs is that there is a pinching (usually from ill fitted boots) that restricts the movement of the tendon through the sheath.

We recommend the following exercises/routines to prevent and/or treat Achilles pain:

- Increase your calf strength. You may notice a trend here. One of the best ways to prevent injury is to build strong muscles. This is why the program emphasizes strength training early in the process long before you start logging significant miles. You must build the foundation before you build the house.

- Proper programming. Build strength then build pace. When you start rucking/running, start low and slow. Build your weight, distance, and pace slowly to give your body time to make the physiological adjustments necessary for high performance. Programs that advocate for long rucks early in the process are inviting injury, training delays, and poor performance.

- Proper fitting boots. Another trend - gear matters. High quality, purpose built, properly fitted gear is essential. The right watch, the right shoes, the right bags. It doesn't have to be expensive, but it absolutely makes a difference. For your boots, you want to be cognizant of the ankle shaft. The boot material, construction technique, and lacing methods can all manipulate the shaft. Look for significant flexing or folding that impedes or presses on the back of the leg/Achilles region. Even gentle pressing that doesn't initially feel bad, can illicit significant pain after a few miles and a few thousand repetitive steps. Cushion heel and cushion shaft socks can also alleviate some pressure. And finally, a good insole that mates well with the heel cup of the boot can provide the proper foot position that reduces friction.

Shin Splints

Medial Tibial Stress Syndrome, or shin splints, is the inflammation of the muscles, tendons, and tissue around the tibia or shin bone. This is most often an overuse injury and is the result of improper conditioning and improper programming. Many new soldiers struggle with shin splints just from the simple act of wearing boots (often for the first time ever) and standing in formation all day. So imagine what a significant load of running and rucking can do to an unconditioned athlete (Ross, 1993).

We recommend the following exercises/routines to prevent and/or treat Shin Splint pain:

- Increase your calf/leg strength. Yes, again. Basics build champions and you must build the foundation before you build the house. The exact same exercises that help with plantar fasciitis will help with shin splints. The good news is that you can get a whole lot of efficiency because the same suite of exercises will cover a multitude of injuries.
- Proper programming. The same principles apply here. Start low and slow and build deliberately. You don't have to worry about this as we've already taken care of the programming. Just monitor your response to the stimuli we program and adjust as required. If you have to slow your progression to accommodate an injury, then so be it.
- Massage. This is one of the injuries that responds well, as opposed to an Achilles injury, to massage as both a preventative measure and a treatment measure. As a preventative measure, massage can help increase the blood flow to the effected muscle but be careful that you aren't massaging so intensely that you're causing damage.

Trapezius Impingement

We cite Trapezius Impingement, but we really mean shoulder injury and dysfunction in general, which often manifests via the trapezius but can more broadly be called Shoulder Impingement Syndrome and is often associated with the scapula. The shoulder is an incredibly complex structure that moves in unique ways and as such is subject to some tremendous forces across these multiple planes. In other words, the shoulder can be delicate, so it should be trained with this in mind. The movements are important and so is the weight management process. In a program where we will be focusing on large loads (especially towards the end), we will be more reserved in our shoulder training weights.

As such, one of the things that we are strongly cautious with shoulder work is within the context of high-intensity timed interval training. In these timed events we find that repetition count is the priority at the sacrifice of proper form. You will often see this phenomenon with kipping pull-ups or overhead press in a CrossFit style MetCon WOD. Men will die for points and the points become the focus, not the form. I've yet to meet a single dedicated multi-year CrossFitter who doesn't have shoulder issues. And the franchise business model and certification process is less rigorous than I would like. This is one of the (many) reasons why I do not recommend CrossFit as a viable SFAS prep tool. So be cautious with your shoulders.

Shoulder impingement most commonly occurs when the rotator cuff, a collection of muscles and tendons that helps your shoulder move, gets "pinched" or compressed. As with our other common injuries, we advocate for building proper musculature to properly support the joint, proper form to avoid injury, and deliberate rehab to recover if injured.

We recommend the following exercises/routines to prevent and/or treat shoulder injury:

- Increase your shoulder strength. We only program Overhead Press as a strength protocol, but if you have a history of injury or some concerns of injury, then you might incorporate some additional exercises. Light weight rotational exercises, lateral lifts, and scapular extensions can all help strengthen the shoulder girdle.
- Proper Form. Form, more than any other variable, should be your focus. Don't let ego get in the way and start piling on weight just because. And control your reps. Your form will degrade as you fatigue, so in weeks with higher rep counts be cognizant of your form and don't be married to the listed range. Bail on a poorly developing rep and let caution win the day. If you try to muscle through a crumbling rep you risk a program-delaying injury.
- Range of Motion. There are a host of shoulder stretches (doorway, cobra, thoracic extension, wall angles, thera-

band work) that can be combined with a solid movement prep (warm-up) routine that will properly prepare your shoulder for the rigors of the workout.

Lower Back

If you intend to make more than a passing attempt at becoming a Special Operator, then you can be nearly assured of lower back issues. Most adult males in the US experience some degenerative disc pain, usually starting around 60 years of age. Our experience is that Special Operators usually experience this pain about 20 years earlier. This makes sense given the inordinate amount of rucking, Airborne operations, cumulative time in body armor, and general intense physical lifestyle. So building a bulletproof back should become a priority. The same principles apply, but with a caveat.

We recommend the following exercises/routines to prevent and/or treat back pain:

- Strength. Deadlift and rows are the cornerstone of a strong back. And proper form is critical, especially given the amount of weight you will eventually be pulling. We can't emphasize proper form enough, particularly with the deadlift. Don't ego lift, train like an athlete.
- Proper programming. This is especially true with ruck programming. Rucking has this mystical connection with back pain. There isn't much literature to support any real connection and I am convinced that the overwhelming majority of this is from improper programming. Too many guys don't train rucking, they go from zero miles and zero weight to a scant 35 pounds and 12 miles and their body simply wasn't conditioned for the shock. Injury is inevitable. We have accounted for this, follow the program.
- Movement Prep. The Back seems to benefit more than any other body part from a good warm-up routine. Taking time to set the conditions for a Back that is primed for

load, movement, and a full range of motion is critical. And it supports maximum performance. We have prepared a comprehensive menu of pre-hab, movement prep, and warm-up exercises and movements that you can choose from to ensure that you get the custom start to your workout that you need. Be in charge of yourself and make certain to do it. Every time.

Mobility

The core of our movement prep effort is mobility. Fluid motion, throughout a full range, with strength and stability in every position. Multi-planar, under load, on unstable ground. This is mobility. Start laying down flat, pop up to hands and knees, swing your legs through to a bear crawl position, flop to a front leaning rest, pike your hips up and walk your hands to your feet, explode to a jump, land in a split squat, and reverse the movement until you're laying flat again. Primal, explosive, dynamic, and strong. Do that ten times and see if you are primed for a productive training session. Mobility is a hallmark of athleticism and it's an investment against injury, particularly in a dynamic and austere environment like SFAS.

There is no official designation or governing body that mandates what mobility sequences are called or what they incorporate in terms of movements and positions. In other words, nobody owns this stuff and there is no standardized naming convention. As such, we will seek to combine descriptive language, common sense, and some narrative to identify the routines that are the most beneficial. We will combine this with the results of a Functional Movement Screening (FMS) that is specifically designed to identify and highlight movement deficiencies. If you have tight shoulders or a weak back, then the FMS will identify it. If you have tight hamstrings or compromised knees, the FMS will tell us. But even if the FMS doesn't show a weakness, and you just sense an imbalance or a feebleness, you can still program specific mobility, flexibility, and strength elements to address it.

You get a vote. This is the part where you get to choose your own adventure. For the strength and endurance programming, you don't get a vote. You have to do the exact lifts and the exact reps at the exact weights that we prescribe. If you knew what you were doing, then you wouldn't have bought the book. For the rucking stuff, you definitely don't get a vote. The collective conventional wisdom on rucking is so poor that it's any wonder anyone gets Selected. So you have to follow the program, to the letter. The only choices you make are against the performance benchmarks that we lay out for each phase. If you meet the benchmark but want an extra week or two to fortify your position, then so be it. But programming is out of your hands. Except for mobility. This is all you.

We will provide a menu of options based on each modality, body part, or deficiency and you will pick and choose which ones you think will satisfy your requirements. You will build, and regularly reassess, your own mobility program. You might build two programs, *Mobility 1* for Strength days and *Mobility 2* for Endurance days. We are going to integrate that program into a movement prep *slash* calisthenics *slash* pre-hab *slash* warm-up routine. It will be become routine. Second nature. You'll do it every day before you lift. You'll do another version before you run or ruck. You decide what stuff needs to be warmed up and to what level so you can execute the program with the intensity that it requires. We'll give you the list and then task you with finding pictures, videos, and tutorials for these and more. There are endless resources with excellent descriptions. It may take a few weeks to get your personal mobility/pre-workout/injury prevention (we'll just call it mobility from here on out) routine as you experiment and adapt to your ever-changing needs. Find the ones that work best you, keep them updated, and stay in tune with your body's feedback. Here is your menu:

MOBILITY, FLEXIBILITY, &
MOVEMENT PREP MENU

I njury Prevention – we are mainly focused on the big 6 that we described earlier, but you can address any lingering concerns here. You can see that we are starting at the ground and moving up the body, but your routine can be whatever preps you best.

- Ball roll for Plantar Fasciitis
- Towel scrunches/roll and towel lifts
- Ankle rotations
- Calf stretch, seated and standing
- Calf Raises, seated and standing
- Banded resistance lunges
- Full ROM Bodyweight squats
- Cossack Squats
- Runners Lunge
- Planks
- Cat/Cow pose
- Childs pose
- Cobra Stretch
- Thread the Needle stretch
- Hyperextensions

- Lumbar Twist
- Doorway stretch
- Thoracic Extension
- Wall angle stretch
- Arm and shoulder circles
- Neck rolls and shrugs

Mobility - We are mainly focused on creating fluid mobility that addresses major joints and hinge points. This should be slow and controlled and can follow or precede the injury prevention work. After injury prevention and mobility work the movement prep and calisthenics can begin.

- Cat/Cow pose
- Spinal Rotation
- Butterfly Sit
- Runners Lunge
- Half Split
- Crescent Lunge
- Lizard Lunge
- Deep Squat
- Pigeon Pose
- Childs Pose
- Cobra Stretch
- Thread the Needle stretch
- Lying Hip Rotations
- Squatting Hip Rotations
- Shinbox Routines
- Piriformis Stretch
- Frog Hip Stretch
- Kneeling Lunge Stretch
- Pike
- Sit Throughs

Calisthenics – He we are addressing some PFA requirements and priming the central nervous system for the pending workout. Push-ups and pull-ups are simply something that we do. There is no drama and there are no specific supersets or drop sets or playing cards. Your warmup will become someone else's workout. When you've done this routine, your body will be ready for the workout. You should aim for multiple sets or round-robin type format.

- Push-ups - Standard, HRPU, Incline/Decline, Diamond, Wide
- Pull-ups - Standard, Fat Bar/Towel, Negatives, Weighted
- Chin-ups
- Dips
- Pike Push-up (shoulders)
- Plank
- Squats
- Split Squats
- Lunges
- Burpees
- Knee Raises
- Box Jumps

NO SHIT, THERE I WAS... MED DROP

S peaking of knowing the difference between being hurt and being injured, I'm reminiscing on one of my most enduring memories of SFAS. As the 3 weeks at Camp Mackall marches along you really see the toll that it takes. Lots of cuts and bruises, endless blisters, and no small number of broken bones. In my class we had a slew of guys with broken feet, and nasty stress fractures in their feet, ankles, and legs.

It's hard to gauge the severity of a stress fracture from just looking at it superficially, but we had guys with deep purple bruises, weird, disfigured joints, and grotesque swelling. I'm no physician, but these dudes were definitely busted up hard. I had a guy on my SFAS team with a broken clavicle. He went so far as to redneck rig a belt to his hip pad on his ruck so he could transfer all the weight onto his healthy shoulder. He got selected.

We weren't so certain about the guys with busted up wheels. They were truly 'walking wounded' but the Cadre are miserly to the extreme with med drops (historically less than 5% of drops...usually ~2%). So these poor guys were hobbling around just refusing to quit. When we were called to formation for the final Long Range Movement, they were standing right there with us. The Company First

Sergeant, a legendary 7th Group Combat Diver named Joe C. (an intimidating physical specimen like all Combat Divers), walks out and calls out a bunch of roster numbers. He ends up calling out the walking wounded, and we were convinced they were going to get a pass on the LRM.

These poor bastards hobble up front with their rucks and Joe says in that deadpan Cadre tone, "Oh good, I just wanted to make sure that ya'll we're still here. Go to the head of the formation and lead the road march." Damn. Zero mercy. We all just sort of stood there in stunned silence. So as the sun sets over the Longleaf Pines, out the gates we go to finish the last march of our stay. One broken foot in front of the other. They made those poor guys go a few miles into the movement before they put them in the ambulance...just far enough to make sure they wouldn't quit. They were standing with us, in casts, at the final Selection formation.

I went on to serve with Joe's son. I was at an event recently and ran into Joe and recounted that story. He's older now, but still fit as hell, and equally as intimidating. He just smiled and chuckled, "Yeah, I remember that." Then he sighed and said, "That was a pretty good class." No higher praise.

YOUR BODY CAN GO SO MUCH FURTHER than you think it can. Learn misery management and the difference between being hurt and being injured, but don't count on anyone else to care. Only your performance matters.

5

NUTRITION, HYDRATION, AND SUPPLEMENTATION

In general, mankind, since the improvement of cookery, eats twice as much as nature requires - Benjamin Franklin

Three Nutritional Truths:

- You cannot out-train a bad diet.
- The Standard American Diet (appropriately abbreviated to SAD) is shockingly bad.
- A good diet is surprisingly easy to develop.

THERE IT IS. The cold, hard facts about *Performance Nutrition*. Nutrition drives performance, proper nutrition is easy, and the typical diet that you likely consume is killing you. There may not be an information environment, save politics, that is more cluttered with half-truths, obfuscation, and chicanery. The message is everything from "Your gut is your second brain," to "You must match your diet to your blood type," all the way to "You can't lose weight because of inherited trauma." Good grief, really? Keto, Paleo, Vegetarian, Vegan, Water Fasting, OMAD, Raw Food, Carnivore, NSNG, Intermittent Fasting, South Beach, Mediterranean, plant-based, alkaline, Macros and Micros...and on and on and on. These things are real, there is some limited scientific evidence for some of the claims, but by and large it is simply more marketing. It keeps the customer base confused and more importantly it keeps them spending.

The reality is much simpler. America is fat. 42% of Americans are obese (CDC, 2021). Think about that number. Almost half of Americans are sloppy fat...that's what obese means. A Body Mass Index greater than 30. It doesn't matter if you're 'big-boned,' if you 'carry it well,' or it 'runs in your family' (maybe your family should do more running). Sloppy fat. It's a national disgrace and it is far more of an existential threat to the Nation and our security than climate change or income inequality or any of the other current causes of virtue. An observant citizen might note that the national decline started when the government got involved in your diet (much the way education in America began its decline when the Federal Department of Education was formed). The USDA Food Pyramid is just bad and the evidence that debunks it is overwhelming. So choose your experts wisely and safely ignore nearly anything that the government tells you. But this fat-epidemic is important to you because the literature is clear that lean body mass is a key predictor of success at SFAS (Farina, et al., Anthropometrics and Body Composition Predict Physical Performance and Selection to Attend Special Forces Training in United States Army Soldiers, 2022). You need to get fast, strong, and lean.

Let's approach performance nutrition with the same eye towards simplicity that we approach everything else. The best way to build strength is *to follow the principle of progressive overload, usually with intense weightlifting, focused on compound movements.* The best way to build rucking performance is *field based progressive load carriage, usually 2-3 times a week, focused on short intense sessions.* And the best way to fuel performance is *balanced whole foods, usually unprocessed, focused on proper protein intake.* That's it. If it's processed, then it's probably bad. If it's not a whole food, then it's likely processed. If you focus on getting proper protein intake, then you'll likely be challenged to eat a bunch of stuff that's bad for you. If your goal is simply to lose weight, then you need to burn more calories than you consume; the standard Calorie In, Calorie Out (CICO) model. You can bend this around and say stupid things like, "What if I only ate Oreo cookies for all of my calories?!" Congratulations, you're now an idiot. Probably a fat idiot.

Let's break down the *balanced whole foods, usually unprocessed, focused on proper protein intake* formula that we advocate. We'll start with balanced whole foods. Balanced means a proper ratio of protein, carbohydrates, and fat at the correct calorie threshold. Before the carnivores jump in to cheer for the flesh, you need carbohydrates to fuel your workouts. They aid in the processing and management of protein. You can certainly manage with very low carbohydrates, but you are likely unnecessarily limiting your performance. You simply need carbs as you will see below. You don't need bread and donuts and excess sugar, but you need carbs. So don't hyper fixate on the macros too much. What you should be more focused on is the processing part (more on this below). Nobody loves a bagel or a nice brioche bun more than me, but that is ultra-processed flour that has been stripped of its nutrients and is essentially just sugar. There is room for simple sugar, but only with purpose and intention. For example, this program will have a bevy of endurance events lasting an hour and longer. Consuming carbohydrates will extend endurance performance, but the physiologic mechanisms for processing carbohydrates will change as the event intensity and duration change. Most forms of carbohydrate can be tolerated up to the 2-hour mark. After 2 hours, focusing on the type of carbohydrate can be important. You should focus on easily digested carbohydrate sources, like glucose, glucose plus fructose, other simple sugars and maltodextrin seem effective. However, when event duration is 2-3 hours, focusing on glucose or maltodextrin, which are rapidly digested and optimizes the absorption of dietary carbohydrates during training. When event duration is expected to extend beyond 2.5 hours, consuming carbohydrates in the form of glucose plus fructose versus glucose alone can enhance your carbohydrate digestion as well as aid in tolerating the higher ingestion rates of carbohydrates needed for these durations. Subsequently, the glucose plus fructose combination will aid in enhancing fluid absorption, may reduce gastrointestinal stress, and can even enhance performance more than when ingesting glucose alone. So carbohydrates are acceptable when they are deliberately programmed with purpose and intention.

The next part of the formula is *usually unprocessed*. Let's be clear, unless you are eating raw fruit that you picked yourself just moments before, then you are eating something that has been 'processed.' Did you wash it? Then it's processed. Did you cut the steak from a larger chunk of meat? Then it's processed. If you are earnestly making this sort of counterargument, then congratulations again, you are an idiot. The USDA defines a processed food as:

> "...one that has undergone any changes to its natural state—that is, any raw agricultural commodity subjected to washing, cleaning, milling, cutting, chopping, heating, pasteurizing, blanching, cooking, canning, freezing, drying, dehydrating, mixing, packaging, or other procedures that alter the food from its natural state." (Harvard School of Public Health, 2023)

For *our* discussion we are talking about processes like adding preservatives, additives, coloring or removing things like fiber. Generally speaking, if it is shelf stable, then it is not good. If it needs artificial coloring to look appealing, then it is not good. This might be a good place to talk about organic and GMO. Whenever we hear the term GMO we immediately think of bad. It has been altered and hacked. If you eat it, it will undoubtedly alter your DNA, right? But most foods that we eat are technically GMO. Another term for GMO might be 'selective breeding.' I plant a crop of tomatoes and save the seeds from the biggest and juiciest tomatoes to replant next season. The weak plants with poor fruit are not selected for next year's crop. After a few seasons, I have selectively planted the best plants with the best fruits. In that process, I have modified the genetic footprint of the crop. Is this dangerous? In and of itself, no. It simply provides me the best plants with the best fruits and ignores the poor performers. That's GMO. There is another GMO. A nefarious GMO. A GMO that alters genetic structures and may produce a higher likelihood of allergic reactions or less resistance to pests. But just saying that GMO = BAD is not correct. Without GMO we wouldn't have corn as we know it. The original corn, or maize, was a low-yield grass that barely resembles the high yield plants that produce massive cobs. So temper your inner-hippie.

The same can be true for organic. This is one of the most abused and misunderstood food terms. There has been a bevy of legislation, first in 1990 and again in 2023, to clarify and enforce the organic moniker. But just because something is organic doesn't mean this it is necessarily better. Technically, human feces and urine fertilizers are organic. Anyone who has some time in Korea can describe for you the joy of a fresh crop of cabbage fertilized this way. Organic does not always mean better. So if you want to ride your high horse through the piss-lettuce fields then just understand what it really means. For *our* formula you must understand the nuance of what processing means for your performance.

The last part of the formula, *focused on proper protein intake*, may present your greatest challenge. There are a few popular formulas to calculate exactly how much protein you should consume each day based on a few variables. They all end up being in the same general ballpark regardless of the formula, so in the interest of simplicity we will use 1 gram of protein per pound of bodyweight. A 150-pound athlete would need 150 grams of protein a day. Simple and easy to calculate. The hard part will be actually eating that much food. Steak, for example, has 7 grams per ounce. So a 12-ounce steak, which is a large hunk of meat, only yields you 84 grams. You should be fully satiated, and you have only gotten roughly half of your requirement. A cup of yogurt gets you about 8 grams of protein. A chicken breast gets you about 50 grams of protein. You need to eat quite a bit of high quality (*balanced whole foods, usually unprocessed*) food in order to get your protein. And don't forget that you need those carbs to get the most of out the protein, too. Suffice it to say, you will likely run out of appetite before you get to your protein goal. Now if you eat a bunch of crap food, like deep fried churros, sodas, full sugar energy drinks, and fast-food slop, you will get your calories, but not your protein. And you need that protein. So in the formula you are working to balance all three elements (*balanced whole foods, usually unprocessed, focused on proper protein intake*) and when you do you will see first-hand how it impacts your performance in both the daily micro and the weekly macro sense.

Hydration

I think the general population is simultaneously under-hydrated and overburdened with hydration accoutrements. You can't swing a dead cat without seeing all manner of bottles, cups, thermoses, flasks, bladders, and jugs (which ironically could easy kill a cat with a quick swing) but they are likely filled with crap. You don't have that luxury. You need to optimize performance, support recovery, enable proper sleep, and aid digestion. So you need to ensure adequate, but not excessive, hydration and maintain an appropriate electrolyte balance. On a "normal" day, ½ ounce per pound of bodyweight per day is adequate (a 200-pound athlete would need 100 ounces). On a hot humid day or high-performance day, an operational athlete might sweat 1-2 liters per hour with some athletes sweating as much as 2-3 liters per hour. You need to monitor how much you are taking in (it's on your daily journal for a reason!). Additionally, the sodium lost through sweat can range from 500-1500 milligrams per liter. Including a sodium source during events aids in reducing electrolyte imbalances and preventing hyponatremia. Hyponatremia is a condition where sodium levels in the blood are abnormally low. This causes nausea, vomiting, fatigue, headache or confusion. On the other end is Hypernatremia, which is an electrolyte problem characterized by increased sodium concentration in the blood. This causes lethargy, confusion, and excessive thirst. Combining sodium appropriately with fluids during events, can also aid in preventing both hypo- and hypernatremia. A loss of just 2% of bodyweight in sweat produces a significant impact in speed and power, cognition and focus, and endurance and recovery. So drink with intent, manage your electrolytes, and track everything.

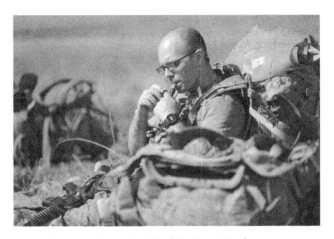

Proper Hydration Is Critical To Sustain Performance

The best way to maintain adequate hydration is to drink early in the morning to get hydrated, sip water throughout the day to maintain hydration, eat mostly whole foods, and in the final three hours of the day limit drinking so you're not up all night emptying your bladder. If you find yourself waking to urinate often then you are likely overhydrating. Similarly, if your mouth is dry at night, it might be mouth breathing not dehydration. What often occurs is that athletes wake up at night feeling parched, they guzzle water as a response, then they have to wake soon thereafter to urinate, then they guzzle water again to relieve their dry mouth and the cycle continues. As you refine your sleep routine (see Chapter 6) you will need to isolate these variables to develop the most ideal structure for you.

Supplementation

If you eat a performance diet consisting of *balanced whole foods, usually unprocessed, focused on proper protein intake,* then you likely don't need much supplementation. I know that this is likely a poor business decision on my part as I'm leaving lots of money on the table for a potential line of TFVooDoo supplements. VooDoo Nootropic Pro-V Hyper-Nitrate Super-Flex Mega-Complex Daily Performance Shake is a money-maker for certain. Let's ask the internet:

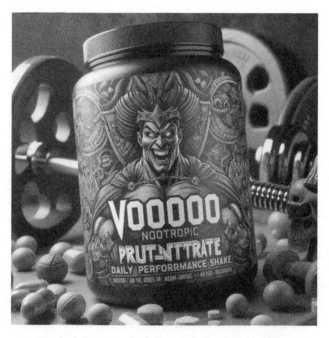

Not bad...lemme rethink this whole supplement thing.
Thank you, AI!

But as discussed earlier, you may struggle to get enough protein. This is particularly true if you are eating from a dining facility on base or on campus with limited options and restricted portions. There are only two supplements that I would endorse, and protein is one of them. So some protein powder supplementation is probably indicated. I would shoot for the 'cleanest' stuff that you can get. The less sugar, flavorings, and additives the better. If you stick with this then there is virtually no risk and no downside for protein supplementation. You may note that the performance journal only asks you to track three nutritional metrics -- total calories, total protein, and hydration. If you want to track all your macros and even your micros, then go ahead. They might give you some insight to really tweak your output, but if you are eating whole foods then you are unlikely to be missing much and protein is the focus.

Creatine is the other supplement that I would endorse. Again, much like protein, there is virtually no health risk from creatine supplementation. It has one of the safest risk profiles of any supplement and the benefits are well documented and not insignificant. Everything from muscle growth to damaged muscle repair to improved cognition (Jaramillo, et al., 2023) (Wu, et al., 2022). Creatine is a performance enhancing drug by every measure. And it's relatively inexpensive. You only need 5 grams a day. No need to calculate load and maintenance doses, just take 5 grams a day. *Not* 5 grams per pound of bodyweight, just 5 grams total. That's it. The benefits are so vast, the risks are so small, and the cost is so low that you should strongly consider supplementation. You get some creatine from meats, but again you are likely to struggle to get enough.

We understand the argument that you shouldn't become dependent on supplements because you won't have access to them at SFAS. There is some merit in this argument as you will indeed not be enjoying any supplements or even decent food while at Camp Mackall. You will mostly eat MREs and only a masochist likes MREs. But we are looking to wring every ounce of efficacy out of our prep and protein and creatine supplementation can help us maintain the intensity and maximize the recovery opportunities. Neither supplement is particularly "potent," in that you are unlikely to *feel* the effects diminishing during the sort of time that you are being assessed. So you don't run much risk of noticeable decreased performance. You will certainly have some negatives, but the benefits during prep far outweigh the potential negatives at SFAS.

We would caution against any stimulant supplements. Caffeine and nicotine are the most prolific, but there are others. We completely understand how effective they are. There is some evidence to suggest that caffeine intake can boost testosterone, but it also simultaneously boosts cortisol (Beaven, et al., 2018). A blast of pre-workout caffeine most definitely enhances your performance. I've tested some stuff that will nearly melt your face. You didn't feel like working out, you popped a pre-workout, and now you can lift a house. Awesome. But I'll give you three drawbacks. The first is you shouldn't become dependent on supplements because you won't have access to them at SFAS. Yes, I'm using my own argument against myself now. It's a win-win. But in this case, if you become dependent on stimulants to *feel* like working out then you are going to struggle significantly when you don't have them. The second drawback is that the stimulants work by, in part, elevating your heart rate. This is going to muddy your data for cardio. Remember, our conditioning work is very heart rate centric. Anything that artificially alters that data is bad. Finally, stimulants will mess with your sleep. You must get your sleep right to get the most out of this process and these stimulants create a nasty cycle of dependency. It's best to simply avoid them.

Finally, let's talk about booze. Nobody loves to blow the froth off a couple of cold ones more than me. Drinking is a central part to team culture. Not necessarily black-out drunk shenanigans. But a nice frosty mug is a relaxing way to finishing out a day on the range or celebrate a mission gone well. There are certainly issues with this, but it is what it is. You need to learn to have a healthy relationship with alcohol, both physically and socially. Nobody will make you drink and there isn't much stigma in being a teetotaler. But the evidence is clear and overwhelming. Alcohol inhibits performance. It delays recovery, reduces effective sleep, and provides no nutritional support. There is no room for booze in your performance nutrition. Save the celebratory cocktail for when you have something to celebrate. Like getting selected.

That is your nutrition plan. The best way to fuel performance is *balanced whole foods, usually unprocessed, focused on proper protein intake.* Stop drinking booze. Drink enough water, with electrolytes, but not too much water. Don't worry about the supplements except for basic protein powder and creatine. If your physical performance is suffering, it's probably because you aren't fueling and resting properly. We have given you broad parameters so that we don't create a bunch of obsessive energy around this topic, but you need to understand just how impactful it can be. You can't out-train a bad diet.

NO SHIT, THERE I WAS...FILL THE TANK

There's always a little urban legend and bad advice that surrounds the frenzied last-minute prep for taking a Physical Fitness Test. The old standard was 2 minutes of push-ups, 2 minutes of sit-ups, and a 2-mile run. Pull-ups weren't added as part of the test until much more recently. Now the test is 2 minutes of hand-release push-ups, plank, 2-mile run, and 6 deadhang pull-ups. So the event has been updated, but the bro-science prep remains much the same.

We had a guy who was convinced that he had to "Fill the Tank" to perform his best. He had some irrational fear that if his hydration level wasn't maxed out that he wouldn't be competitive. Back in the day, some classes used the PT test as a screening tool to cull class sizes, so you very much felt the pressure to perform, or you might not even get to go to Camp Mackall. This pressure was particularly acute at the end of the alphabet. Classes were organized alphabetically by last name, so if you were at the end of the line, you might find yourself facing a grader that had already met his quota. No matter how many push-ups you did, he wasn't going to count any more than 31, leaving you alone with your performance drop.

So "Fill the Tank" guy was keen to give himself every advantage that he could. In his mind, this meant tripling the concentration of his Oral Rehydration Salts and using warm water to speed the absorption. But what really happened is that he filled his tank with a potent warm tea laxative. An already nervous Candidate, a jittery stomach, and a nice chug of warm salty water sloshing around in his belly.

He seemed to manage the push-ups and sit-ups without too much issue. Although I wouldn't have wanted to be the guy holding his feet for the sit-ups. That's the Splash Zone. Come run time you could see the worry on his face. His confidence in his farts was low. He was feeling the pressure, in more ways than one. We used to run the test on an outdoor track in heats and it was always a little crowded. The pack thinned pretty quickly as the rabbits set the pace and the "tankers" brought up the rear.

As the faster guys finished and congregated around the finish line you could bear witness to those last minutes of desperation. Fill The Tank guy was particularly desperate. It was clear that his strategy wasn't working, and he had overplayed his hand. He was definitely trying hard, but not at running. He had that desperate cheek-clenched shuffle that usually follows taco and beer night. He was moving as fast as he could, but his distress was obvious.

The grader was calling out the time and Fill the Tank had his mark. It was go time. So he released the brakes and dropped the hammer. As he was closing in on the finish line, he also released his tank. This is when we wore the grey PT uniform, so no black shorts to mask the overflow. He slid across the finish line with a bowel full of warm ORS tea sliding down his backside.

The tank was empty. At last.

HE MISSED THE CUTOFF SCORE, but I don't think that he would have lasted much past that anyway. He was a marked man, in more ways than one. So just stick to sipping regular water. Leave that hocus-pocus bro-science out.

6

SLEEP AND RECOVERY

What stands in the way becomes the way. - Marcus Aurelius

Whenever an aspiring Candidate reaches out to get help with their prep, they are always looking to tweak a lift, a running routine, or a rucking technique. These are the foundations of performance after all, correct? I always hear them out and let them make their pitch. They are usually fairly precise in their assessment and come ready with lots of data. They can list times and weights and paces and the various sundry of data points that one might expect. I pause, and then ask about their sleep and diet. Their diet is almost always trashy food, poorly measured, and washed down with lots of booze and energy drinks. We've already covered this at some length in Chapter 5. The sleep is even worse. Sleep is the best stress relief, the best immune booster, the best hormone regulator, the best emotional stabilizer, and the absolute best recovery tool available to you. What is even more frustrating is that proper sleep isn't wildly aspirational. It is simple little tasks, consistently executed, with immense and immediate performance gains. Get your sleep in order and your training will soon follow.

Just like you can't out-train a bad diet, you can't out-train bad sleep either. And the links between diet and sleep can't be ignored. Sleep deprivation, even moderate deprivation, is incredibly unhealthy if not downright dangerous. The links between sleep deprivation and brain function and systemic physiology are numerous. It impacts your metabolism, appetite regulation, and your immune, hormonal, and cardiovascular systems (Medic, Wille, & Hemels, 2017). Yes, the quality of your sleep impacts your run and ruck performance.

In the military we wield sleep deprivation as a regular training tool, and we often authorize the least qualified and foolish to weaponize it. The result is that we build a culture of ambivalence about sleep, and we misunderstand its impact. This tool (sleep restriction/sleep deprivation) will inevitably be used against you during SFAS. While this will largely be outside of your control, this is in part why it is so vital to get your sleep squared away in your train up. A healthy sleep schedule and sleep physiology is significantly more resilient toward acute sleep disturbances or disruptions, allowing you to maintain your performance for longer.

The quality of your sleep is a great deal governed by the choices you make throughout the day. Stuff that you do in the morning can impact how you respond later that night. What you eat, and when, impacts sleep quality. Your environment, all of it, impacts the quality of your sleep. All of these are things that you control. There is nothing random about this. Your body has a natural internal clock, known as the circadian rhythm, that effects sleep, hunger, hormonal, and stress responses.

It is most effected by light and dark, but there is much we can do to support its normal functioning (Reddy, Reddy, & Sharma, 2023). In a moment we will cover light as a part of your specific sleep environment, but let's cover light as a component of habit, routine, and preparation for sleep first. In order to get the sort of maximally restive (aka restorative) sleep that you need to sustain performance for this program you can't just prep for sleep in the brief moments before you lay down at night. You need to set conditions for night success starting the moment that you wake up. In order to help reestablish your circadian cycle, you should get early morning sunlight within 30-60 minutes of waking. If you're still doing your sleep math this may conflict with your schedule, especially in the winter with the late sunrise. If you're getting up at 5 AM and the sun doesn't rise until 7 AM, then you're not making that 30-60 minute window. So endeavor to catch the sun as soon as possible. Literally just go outside and let the sun shine in your face. Not through a window or a windshield, but directly in the face. Don't stare at the sun but get 10 minutes of direct sunlight within 30-60 minutes of arising. Get another 10-minute session of sunlight just before the sun sets as well for maximal benefit, but the morning session is non-negotiable (Gooley, 2017). In the absence of sunlight, try to get bright artificial light as a replacement. Bookending your day with sunlight serves as a definitive cue for your circadian rhythm. This ensures that your body secretes the necessary hormones to maximize alertness during periods of wakefulness and secretes melatonin at appropriate times to promote better sleep.

We will cover the power of routines and the innate human need for them in Chapter 9, but let's focus on this specific routine here. First is the routine timing, both in regularity and duration. The literature is clear that 7-8 hours is optimum, but perhaps even more important is the go to bed and wake up times (Sletten, et al., 2023). Maintaining consistency is key. Go to bed at the same time and wake up at the same time. Weeknights, weekends, and holidays. Stay consistent. If you have to wake up early for work, then you have to go to bed early.

Do some math here; if 7-8 hours is optimal and you have to be up at 5 AM, then you have to be in bed at 9 or 10 PM. Are you a 'night owl?' Do you like to stay up late? Not anymore. You're a professional tactical athlete and you need your sleep. If you have high sleep latency, it takes you a long time to fall asleep, then you might need even more time. Not only does one's latency impact the calculus of establishing bed times and wake times, but the fact that people do not sleep with 100% efficiency is also impactful. In fact, healthy ranges of sleep efficiency are roughly between 80-95%. So if we are trying to protect 7-8 hours of sleep per night, we need to factor in additional time that is lost due to natural nighttime awakenings. And remember, the literature is clear that consistency is more important than duration, so if you get to bed late (because you were undisciplined) you don't get to sleep in late. You're just delaying the problem and hurting your chances for a good night's sleep the following night. Go to bed at the same time, wake up at the same time, get 7-8 hours a night, and don't stay up late for something that you wouldn't get up early for.

Note: You might be doing a lot of margin math at this point, and you will likely be struggling to reconcile all of the requirements. They are often conflicting or at the least very obstructive. We will provide a Perfect Week to illustrate how you might negotiate this program in practicum, but there are certainly sacrifices to be made. This is a demanding lifestyle, and it will require sacrifice.

Use napping sparingly. If you do nap, limit it to less than 90 minutes. The 'ideal' nap length to restore alertness and cognitive function is ~26 minutes, which has been established through NASA astronaut protocols (Rosekind, et al., 1995). There are some benefits for performance, cognitive functioning, and alertness, but these are most pronounced in those subjects that already have regular sleep/wake schedules (Milner & Cote, 2009). Think of napping as a supplement, rather than a resolution to a larger problem. This is less applicable during the more structured train up time, but more likely to be implemented during 'hurry up and wait' time during SFAS. And the literature is very clear that while there are clear benefits to napping, those benefits are significantly amplified when measured after a full night's sleep, to the point that I would assess that napping as almost wasted time. If you are looking for the best sleep, then get a full night versus a nap (Schalkwijk, et al., 2017).

What you eat and when you eat it also impacts your sleep quality. Caffeine, a central ingredient in energy drinks, should be avoided whenever possible and certainly in the afternoons. This means that if you normally schedule your workouts in the afternoon and you partake in pre-workout supplementation then you will likely be impacting your sleep quality. As a result, you wake up tired, so you look for stimulants to stay alert. These stimulants negatively impact your sleep that night and you awaken not fully rested. Caffeine half-life is ~6 hours. This means that only half of the dose of caffeine you ingested have left your system at the 6-hour mark. So at minimum, we should curb caffeine usage 6 hours before our planned bedtime, if not earlier, especially tied to our mg dosage. The vicious cycle repeats and you never fully recover, you never realize the performance gains that you need, and your hormones actually end up damaging your advances. When you do get up in the morning, after you get your 10 minutes of early morning sun, you should delay any caffeine intake for 60-90 minutes. When you consume caffeine immediately on waking you also spike cortisol levels (Lovallo, et al., 2005). There is a documented testosterone boost for exercise when supplemented with caffeine, but there is also a cortisol spike so the resultant testosterone to cortisol ratio may not be worth the opposing catabolic effects (Beaven, et al., 2018).

Your takeaway from this discussion should be that caffeine is not just some benign supplement that gives you a good zap of energy when you wake up and when you head to the gym. It is a powerful stimulant that has deep impacts on your hormones and sleep. Use it both sparingly and intentionally. I would also caution against too much sleep supplementation like Magnesium Threonate, Magnesium Bisglycinate, Apigenin, Theanine, or Melatonin. We think that it's even more important for people to use caution with the quality of the supplements. As we know, the FDA does not regulate supplements since they fall under the performance enhancement space. As a result, many supplements you will find are not only poorly formulated, but inaccurate in their dosages and even contents. Steer towards only 3rd-party certified brands to ensure you are getting what they claim. We recommend none at all if tenable, but sleep is so critical to your performance and recovery that once you have exhausted and perfected your sleep hygiene and sleep routine, I could see an argument to supplement if you aren't reaching 7-8 solid hours of sleep per night.

Alcohol should be avoided for a number of reasons, but specifically for sleep quality. Alcohol is a commonly used "over the counter" sleep aid. In healthy adults, alcohol decreases sleep latency, consolidates and increases the quality and quantity of deep restorative sleep, but only during the first half of the night. Sleep is disrupted during the second half of the night, and this is when your most restorative sleep usually occurs (Thakkar, Sharma, & Sahota, 2015). You are robbing Peter to pay Paul. Additionally, insufficient sleep adversely impacts dietary intakes, meaning you are more likely to make poor food choices when sleep deprived. Whole diets rich in fruits, vegetables, legumes, and other sources of dietary tryptophan and melatonin have been shown to predict favorable sleep outcomes (Zuraikat, Wood, Barragán, & St-Onge, 2021).

Next, we will cover your sleep setting - the noise, light, temperature, and touch – that support proper sleep. You want to create a maximally permissive sleep environment. Many of us have to contend with communal (barracks), quasi-communal (roommates), or intimate communal (spouses) sleeping accommodations so we might have some compromises here, but we should endeavor to manipulate these to our benefit as much as possible. Our first variable is temperature. Thermoregulation is strongly linked to the mechanism regulating sleep and may be the single most important variable, so your thermal environment is a key determinant of sleep quality (Okamoto-Mizuno & Mizuno, 2012). The body needs to drop in temperature by 1-3 degrees to fall and stay asleep effectively (Harding, Franks, & Wisden, 2020). Body temperature increases are one reason you wake up. You can manipulate your body temp, counterintuitively, by taking a warm bath or shower before bedtime. The heating of your skin triggers the body to send warm blood from the core (Haghayegh, Khoshnevis, Smolensky, Diller, & Castriotta, 2019). Even simply warming your hands and feet can have an impact on deep sleep and sleep latency (the time between when you lay down and when you actually fall asleep) (Krauchi, Werth, & Wirz-Justice,

1999). Most literature puts the ideal sleeping temperature between 65-68 degrees Fahrenheit. If this is a tough sell for your spouse or room-mates, this is where the warm bath or shower is most critical. What you wear to sleep in matters. Lightweight and loose-fitting clothes are best as they allow for your body to thermoregulate naturally. Sleeping naked is the ultimate manifestation of this tactic. Barrel-Chested Freedom Fighting Commando is truly a lifestyle!

Our next environmental variable is light. We know that exposure to artificial light at night can deeply impact the quality of sleep (Cho, et al., 2015). As such, we should endeavor to make the room we sleep in as dark as possible. Once you start looking deliberately, you'll be surprised how much light spills into your room. Phone chargers and the phones themselves, clocks, smart watches, speakers, routers and modems, and even unused charging cables with LED tips or power strips. Perform a light-hygiene survey of your sleep quarters and look for all of these sources. Be hyper-meticulous and cover every source with some gaffers tape or stickers. Wear a sleep mask. Get heavy blackout curtains and create a cocoon of darkness to minimize any lights that might influence your circadian cycle. Avoid bright lights in the evening, including using your phone. Curbing device usage about an hour before bed is the goal. Lights signal your brain to alert, so lights at night send stimuli signals to your brain and hinder your natural circadian cycle. We don't need to limit our evening routines to candlelight or tactical red lights, but darker is better.

Touch refers to the comfort component. Soft, loose, or no night clothes, soft linens, and an appropriately firm mattress and pillows. I can't emphasize enough the value of a good mattress. You are going to be putting your body through an absolute wringer. If you're curling up on some second-rate foam, you're not going to recover effectively. You should be spending about a third of your prep sleeping, so invest in your recovery. Even if you sleep in the barracks, you can get a quality mattress topper than can enhance the prison mat they provide for you. The same goes for pillows. Spend a little bit on a quality mattress and pillows and you will get that return on your investment. Sheets and blankets should get some deliberate attention as well. Your blanket system is a central node to your thermal regulation. If you can seamlessly add or subtract layers during the night without fully awakening, then all the better. And comfortable sheets don't have to be expensive. Keep your linens, night clothes, and pillows well laundered and for less than a few hundred dollars you can develop a solid system that enhances your recovery, not inhibits it.

The final environmental factor is noise. Communal quarters complicate this significantly, but there is clear evidence that sleep disturbances are associated with health deterioration, and it has been proven that nocturnal noise pollution significantly impairs sleep (Halperin, 2014). We recommend a white noise machine or even a fan. The literature strongly indicates that white noise significantly improves sleep quality (Ebben, Yan, & Krieger, 2019). In the vein of white noise, are pink noise devices. These work foundationally the same as white noise, helping to block out the bumps in the night that alter our brain, but also are designed to induce brain waves that shift us into deeper, more restorative sleep. So with a little bit of due diligence and a little bit of effort, you can manipulate the light, noise, touch, and temperature in your sleep quarters to create a permissive sleep environment that enables recovery. You're going to need all of the best quality sleep that you can get. Your sleep environment (as defined by light, noise, temperature, and touch), your nutrition and supplementation, and your daily routine (napping and light exposure) all combine to create the conditions for sleep.

The final element is your sleep routine, that is the specific things you do in the hours leading up to going to bed, that set the conditions for proper restive sleep. Again, we will harness the power of routine and habit. What you are essentially doing is programming a Pavlovian response to fall asleep quickly, enter deep sleep, and awaken at optimum alertness. It starts with light. As the evening progresses start controlling your lights. Avoid bright lights and avoid screen time. The specific blue light of phone and tablet screens decreases the quality and duration of sleep (Silvani, Werder, & Perret, 2022). Keep lights low and avoid using your phone. Avoid food in general, and caffeine specifically, in the last 3-4 hours before bed. Pick low energy activities like light stretching, reading, or journaling. Spend some time organizing yourself for the following day. Lay out your clothes, pack any bags, and prepare your food. If you are fully prepared for the next day, it will clear your mind of that cognitive load. Reserve your bed for only sleeping if possible. Do your reading and journaling in another room so that you condition yourself so that when you lay down in your bed, you go to sleep.

Your environment is set with low lights, cool temperature, white noise, and soft sheets and night clothes. Your mattress is just right, and you have layers of blankets to peel off or add as you manage your thermoregulation throughout the night. You've had your warm bath or shower, you've cleared your mind with your journaling, and you're ready to lay down. Your mind is clear. But not overly alert because it's been several hours since you ate and almost half a day or more since you had any caffeine. You were up early that day, got your early morning sun, and had an intense workout so you are ready to begin your recovery. Off to la-la land you go, right on time, in the same 30-minute window that you go to bed every night. A perfect night of sleep. When you wake up the next morning, you'll do it all again. Consistency is key and you need to rest. You've earned it.

Non-Sleep Deep Rest

If you don't get the sleep that you need you can employ a technique called Non-Sleep Deep Rest (NSDR). NSDR is a mindfulness, meditation, and relaxation technique that is sometimes referred to as *yoga nidra* that mimics the effects of falling asleep without actually sleeping. It can be an effective stop gap measure for days that life gets in the way. NSDR works by slowing down brain wave frequencies, mirroring the patterns observed during slow-wave sleep (SWS). Slow-wave sleep, also known as deep sleep, is one of the four stages of sleep and represents the third phase of non-rapid eye movement sleep (non-REM sleep). During this stage, delta waves dominate the electroencephalogram (EEG), a device used to measure brain activity (Huberman, 2023). NSDR tricks your brain into being rested and you can enjoy some element of alertness. You likely aren't getting the recovery that you need long term, but as a short-term sustainment tool it can be useful to get you through the day. It will also be helpful in SFAS when you definitely won't be getting enough sleep. A discrete NSDR session can give you the mental clarity that you need during that next critical assessment, without too much scrutiny.

A deliberate sleep environment supported by good nutrition and light habits, that is supplemented by NSDR will be critical, probably tied neck and neck with nutrition, to maintaining high performance. If you feel like you need an energy drink, which will inevitably screw up your sleep later, try an NSDR session. When you start to reach plateaus or are struggling with maintaining consistency, look to your sleep first. Everyone likes to focus on the lifting and the running and the rucking and forget about sleeping and eating for performance. Before you start adding extra exercises or workout sessions, dial in your sleep to the finest degree possible and give it a week to start taking effect. Then look at your diet, which as we described is intimately interconnected to your sleep. Once you have those two dialed in you can start monkeying with the 'fun' stuff. Basics build champions. Sleep like your life depends on it.

NO SHIT, THERE I WAS...CALLING ON THE ALMIGHTY

The Army uses sleep deprivation as a common tool for inducing "combat stress." It's seen as a simple and low-cost method to induce the fog of war and simulate combat conditions. For the record, whenever I've deployed, I've gotten excellent sleep so I'm not certain how this theory works. But the utility is apparent. And if the Army does it because it's hard, then when SF does it, we're going to make it harder. SFAS is a prime example of this. You will get very limited, closely monitored sleep during most of SFAS. You get a few hours a night, you have insufficient calories, and your work output is tremendous. So sleep is a constant need, and you are extremely fatigued.

Because you are so exhausted, you end up falling asleep at the drop of a hat. It's not like Ranger School fatigue, which is sort of a grinding exhaustion. The SFAS collapse is very sudden. One minute you're fighting for your life under the Sandman, and the next minute your team is taking a break on the side of the road and you're out cold. It doesn't stalk you, kidnap you, and hoist you above a quicksand pit for slow demise. It hits you like a 300 Win Mag right in the head. You go from fully conscious and engaged to passed out in less than a minute.

Candidates get creative with the excuses when they get caught sleeping. It was a common tactic when we were in the barracks to slide under your bed and tuck your fingers in between the mattress and the spring frame and make it look like you were tucking in your sheets for a squared away rack. You could catch a pretty decent combat nap in this configuration. This is a tactic that you learn well in Basic Training. It might gain you a few precious seconds of warning from an approaching Drill Sergeant. The problem at SFAS is that you don't get issued sheets and a blanket. You sleep in your fart sack (sleeping bag) so there is no rack to square away. Cadre are like ninjas in the barracks, and they will often walk through stealthily unannounced and catch Candidates sleeping.

Out in the field, say during Team Week, there is little camouflage to conceal your combat naps. Especially when they hit you like sniper fire and you do nothing to prepare your hide site beforehand. So you need a cover story for when you inevitably get caught napping. There is the always chambered excuse of flat denial. "I wasn't sleeping, Sarn't." "Yes, yes you were. You actually have a drool mark on your shirt." A lot of guys like to call on the Almighty in these times of need. When they get caught in a quiet moment of repose they will respond with, "I wasn't sleeping, Sarn't. I was just saying a prayer."

Candidates think they've discovered a secret loophole of religious freedom. "Nobody can penalize me for exercising my religious beliefs," they think. There are no Grey Men at SFAS, all the rules matter all the time, and Cadre have seen it all. About 3,500 guys a year go through SFAS, so Cadre are well-versed in your barracks lawyer nonsense. After a few rounds of call to prayer, Cadre will simply respond with, "Oh, you were saying a prayer, were you? Well, you'd better pray that you get Selected, because if I catch you sleeping again, you're going to need some divine intervention!"

Do your NSDR with your eyes open. Or God help ya!

7

MENTAL RESILIENCY AND COGNITION

The world will ask you who you are and if you don't know the world will tell you. - Jung

Your brain exists for two purposes; to keep you safe and to keep you comfortable. Safe and comfortable. That's the priority. It engages in a lot of different processes, but ALL of them, ultimately happen in order to serve the primal programming towards safety and comfort. As our resident Cognitive Performance Specialist Nate likes to say "Keep the meat-sack alive. Keep the meat-sack in some semblance of balance." I think that it's safe to say that there is very little about your SFAS prep, Selection itself, or your greater Special Forces endeavor that is either particularly safe or comfortable. This is a difficult position for you. You need to build a strong relationship with your brain. You are going to need your brain, at its peak performance, during your entire stay at Camp Mackall. Working against your primal instinct can be challenging. And to make matters worse, we have carefully crafted the assessment environment to be as difficult as possible. It will seem as dangerous and uncomfortable as you could imagine. No performance feedback, precariously constructed junkyard apparatuses, and long solo treks through the woods at night. Your brain will struggle when conditions are perfect. When we throw in a lingering blister or a twisted ankle you will really see the lesser prepared stumble mightily. God help those people if it rains. I always simply called this stuff cognitive load, but Nate says it much more precisely: "Managing all the internal noise that your mind generates can quickly become an overwhelming task. That is, IF we haven't developed the appropriate relationship with our mind." I like this much more because it conjects that you have some agency over the process. It's not just something that happens to you. You can control it.

And this is just the baseline position. Survival mode if you will. This is the level of just getting by and just getting by isn't enough to get selected. You need some strategies to manage this cognitive load (or as Nate notes, "Manage the various internal landmines to reduce cognitive load"), develop excess cerebral processing capacity, and be able to effectively engage with the task at hand. You can't just survive; you need to thrive. This prep program is specifically designed to make you engage with maximum physical intensity. Take, for example, rucking. Rucking sucks. If you are some sort of masochist, you might be able to convince yourself and others that you enjoy rucking. But you don't. Nobody normal enjoys it. Now we're not talking about some 15-pound, 15-minute mile, trail shoe-wearing jaunt along the Riverwalk. This isn't the social rucking that folks like to trot out as evidence of hardiness (like those Spartan racers who equate those 5K fun runs to the Bataan Death March). We're talking about military rucking. In the military, we can suck the fun out of skydiving, scuba diving, and shooting with ease. So we can certainly take the fun out of an already miserable activity like rucking. As such, what most of us do is purposefully insulate ourselves from the misery. When given the opportunity during a ruck, virtually everyone likes to pop in their earbuds and listen to music or a podcast in order to distract themselves from this misery. They are intentionally turning their brain off, a dissociative approach, in the exact moment that they need to engage their brains deliberately. The literature is clear here. In sum, do not separate your mental prep and your physical prep. Every important decision that you make at SFAS you will make with a ruck on your back. If you are training to desynchronize the physical and mental, then you will not be adequately prepared to engage in the assessment environment. Nate states it well: "There is a time and place for being a 'big, dumb, animal'. That time and place is less common than you might think during SFAS. We need to always remain vigilant to both our external AND internal environment in order to maximize our performance." Perfectly stated.

Let's put this concept in context and expand on a discussion that we previously explored in RUSU in terms of managing cognitive load during Land Navigation. Land Nav at SFAS is unique in the DoD in that it is one of the few places where Land Nav is done with a ruck on your back. And it's a heavy ruck, usually tipping the scale around 70 pounds or more. And there are few tasks that require more cognitive engagement than Land Nav. Just a few moments of poorly managed cognition and you are hopelessly lost, you can't find your weapon, and your ruck is submerged deep in a draw. What usually happens is that poorly prepared Candidates will fight to prioritize cognition for proper navigation, but the persistence of the ruck misery overpowers that cognition. Nate had a particularly noteworthy point that has escaped me until recently. People lose their minds during land navigation particularly. Not only does the physical toll make them less likely to pause and engage their brain, but the mere idea of a time hack is known to shift us from choosing to reacting. Typically, the first thing to go when performing under a time pressure is our willingness to plan. This is exceptionally problematic when developing and adhering to an effective route plan, which is critical in land navigation. If you want to keep moving, then you don't have a choice. Similarly, your brain is the most calorie consuming organ in your body, but because you have a ruck on your back and you need to keep moving, your brain is in a knife fight with your legs, back, and core. So, cognition suffers. Unless you take deliberate steps to train for this exact condition. We will train for these conditions specifically and add logic games, riddles, and cognition into many of our conditioning workouts. It's a simple step, with a huge return on investment but it's not necessarily a primary tool. Nate advises that focusing on more general logic and problem-solving type exercises is more directly relevant to the types of thinking one must be able to execute within SFAS and later as an Operator. In addition, we will include observation exercises that force the individual to maintain environmental/situational awareness, since that is essential to demonstrating adaptability and psychological flexibility.

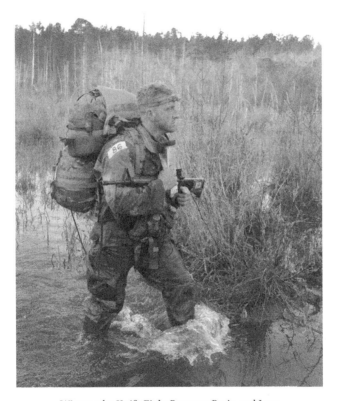

Witness the Knife Fight Between Brain and Legs

When I first met Dr. Sean Burkhardt, it was through his research in the neuroscience behind the Green Berets. Sean is a DC, a Doctor of Chiropractic medicine, so his medicine is manual medicine. Manual medicine can include hands-on work on joints and tissues.

But I find that D.C. are often more holistic and while they must complete training as residents in the specialty they choose and they also must pass the same licensing exam before they can treat people, they tend to have less invasive treatment and eschew pharmaceuticals. They look for the interconnectedness of conditions. You may recall that I described Operational Fitness as interconnected. You may also note that we have established a fairly foreseeable pattern of repeated basic tenets. Fundamentals and foundations and frameworks. Axioms and essentials and context. It is systems thinking in action.

Sean was treating these SF guys with late career physical issues and wondering what it was that was driving them to push themselves like they were. He was interested in learning the mindset. It is here that Sean really catches his stride. He is a *Neuro-Performance* expert. He did what he does, he traced the injury to its origins and along the way he discovered the neuroscience behind the ARSOF Attributes. I am extremely well-versed in the whole SFAS process and particularly so in the factor analysis of assessing the ARSOF Attributes. It is the very core of the Assessment process. Everyone thinks Selection is about the physical, but it is far more about assessing these Attributes. And Sean has examined and explained how the mind and body connection manifest to present these Attributes. I want to share a portion of a paper that Sean authored, and I want to present it with as few interruptions and edits as possible. I want to do this because I want you to see how he interprets the science behind the Attributes. As a Subject Matter Expert on SFAS I was struck by how insightful his analysis is. He wrote this after months of research, including reading *Ruck Up Or Shut Up*, but before we teamed up deliberately. And he nailed it. I have always counseled prospective Candidates that they can't hide who they truly are. SFAS will break you down and the brain will simply do what the brain does. There truly are no Grey Men, and Dr. Burkhardt explains the how behind the why.

The Neuroscience Behind Core Attributes for Special Forces Assessment and Selection Candidates

IN THE DEMANDING world of Special Forces Assessment and Selection, the journey to getting your Green Beret extends far beyond the realms of rigorous physical training. It delves deep into the cognitive and psychological makeup of an individual. This chapter is dedicated to unraveling the complex neuroscience behind the core attributes essential for candidates undergoing assessment and selection in special operations. Here, we explore how these attributes, far from being abstract qualities, are deeply rooted in specific neural networks and brain functions necessary to develop the mental fortitude to succeed.

The preparation for selection in special operations involves a crucial cognitive piece that revolves around innate attributes and traits. These attributes are not just personality markers but are intricately linked to specific brain regions and functions. Through a thorough evaluation process, candidates can gain profound insights into their strengths and weaknesses concerning these key attributes. Understanding this neuroscientific basis is vital, as it allows for tailored training that enhances both cognitive abilities and physical performance. The rationale is clear: the brain regions responsible for these core attributes are inextricably linked to one's ability to focus, make decisions under pressure, and execute tasks with precision.

In the context of the Army Special Operations Forces (ARSOF), these attributes are not just desirable qualities but are central to the ethos and effectiveness of these elite units. Developed and emphasized by the United States Army John F. Kennedy Special Warfare Center and School, the Special Operations Center of Excellence, these attributes form the benchmark for the selection and development of special operation soldiers. They are not merely guidelines but are foundational to the very identity and capability of ARSOF personnel.

This section will delve into each of these attributes, exploring their neuroscientific underpinnings and their impact on the cognitive and physical aspects of a Special Forces candidate. From integrity and adaptability to decisiveness and professionalism, we will dissect how these qualities are manifested in the brain, and how targeted training can enhance these attributes to meet the demanding standards of special operations. The goal is to provide a comprehensive understanding that preparation for Special Forces is a holistic endeavor, encompassing both the mind and body in a seamless continuum of excellence.

Let's delve into the brain areas and networks associated with traits crucial for Special Forces candidates, such as integrity, courage, perseverance, adaptability, personal responsibility, professionalism, physical and mental capability, and being a team player. I'll also provide examples of how these traits manifest in the context of SFAS.

ARSOF Core Attributes from USAJFKSWCS

1. **Integrity - Being trustworthy and honest; acting with honor and unwavering adherence to ethical standards.**
    - Brain Areas: Prefrontal Cortex (PFC), Temporal Lobes, Amygdala, Anterior Cingulate Cortex (ACC)
    - *Special Forces Example:* A candidate demonstrating integrity might refuse to cheat during a navigation exercise, despite being under immense pressure and fatigue.

2. **Courage - Acting on own convictions despite consequences; is willing to sacrifice for a larger cause; not paralyzed by fear of failure.**
    - Brain Areas: Amygdala, Ventromedial, and Dorsolateral PFC.
    - *Special Forces Example:* A candidate shows courage by leading a team through a high-risk scenario in training, managing fear, and making decisive choices under threat.

· · ·

3. <u>Perseverance - Working toward an end; has commitment; physical or mental resolve; motivated; gives effort to the cause; does not quit.</u>

- Brain Areas: Anterior Cingulate Cortex (ACC), Insular Cortex, and Basal Ganglia.

- *Special Forces Example:* A candidate exhibits perseverance by continuing to push through a grueling land navigation evolution, despite physical exhaustion and a heavy ruck.

4. <u>Adaptability - Possessing the ability to maintain composure while responding to or adjusting one's thinking and actions to fit a changing environment; the ability to think and solve problems in unconventional ways; the ability to recognize, understand, and navigate within multiple social networks; the ability to proactively shape the environment or circumstances in anticipation of desired outcomes.</u>

- Brain Areas: Orbitofrontal Cortex, Hippocampus, and Amygdala

- *Special Forces Example:* Adaptability is shown when a candidate quickly adjusts to a sudden change in mission/leadership parameters during a field exercise, effectively altering strategies to meet new objectives.

5. <u>Personal Responsibility - Being self-motivated and an autonomous self-starter; anticipates tasks and acts accordingly; takes accountability for his actions.</u>

- Brain Areas: PFC, ACC, Amygdala, Insular Cortex.

- *Special Forces Example:* A candidate taking personal responsibility might acknowledge and learn from a mistake during a tactical exercise, rather than blaming external factors.

. . .

6. **Professionalism - Behaving as a standard-bearer for the regiment; has a professional image, including a level of maturity and judgment mixed with confidence and humility; forms sound opinions and makes own decisions; stands behind his sensible decisions based on his experiences.**

- Brain Areas: PFC, Temporal-Parietal Junction (TPJ), ACC, Amygdala.

- *Special Forces Example:* Professionalism is evident when a candidate consistently demonstrates respect for cadre and peers, adheres to protocol, and maintains composure in high-pressure situations.

7. **Capability - Maintaining physical fitness, including strength and agility; has operational knowledge; able to plan and communicate effectively.**

- Brain Areas: Motor Cortex, Cerebellum, PFC, ACC, Limbic System.

- *Special Forces Example:* This trait is vital for enduring physically demanding tasks like ruck marches and mentally challenging tasks like tactical decision-making under stress.

8. **Team Player - Possessing the ability to work on a team for a greater purpose than himself; dependable and loyal; works selflessly with a sense of duty; respects others and recognizes diversity.**

- Brain Areas: PFC, Mirror Neuron System, TPJ.

- *Special Forces Example:* A candidate who excels as a team player might effectively coordinate with others during a team week challenge, showing empathy and understanding towards team members' strengths and weaknesses.

CONTEXTUALIZING **with Neuroscience**

- These traits involve complex neural networks, the descriptions above are meant to shed light on the complex neurological processes however, not an all-inclusive list. This indicates that a range of cognitive and emotional processes are present during the activation of these attributes. All are essential for a successful Special Forces candidate.

- The development of these traits can be influenced by training and experience, highlighting the brain's plasticity.

- The Special Forces assessment process tests these traits in extreme conditions, simulating the stress and unpredictability of real-world operations.

In summary, Special Forces candidates must possess a unique combination of physical and mental traits, underpinned by specific brain areas and networks. These traits are not only innate but can be cultivated and enhanced through rigorous training and experience.

Specific roles of the prefrontal cortex, temporal lobes and the amygdala concerning the trait of integrity, especially in the context of a Special Forces Assessment and Selection (SFAS) candidate.

PREFRONTAL CORTEX (PFC)

Decision-Making and Moral Judgment: The PFC, particularly areas like the ventromedial and dorsolateral PFC, is heavily involved in decision-making processes that incorporate moral and ethical judgment. For an SFAS candidate, this means consistently making choices that align with the high moral standards expected in Special Forces, even under extreme stress or when faced with morally ambiguous situations.

Impulse Control and Long-Term Planning: The PFC is crucial for inhibiting impulsive behaviors and focusing on long-term goals over immediate gratification. An SFAS candidate must exhibit the ability to control impulses and make decisions that benefit the mission and team, even if they require personal sacrifice or delayed rewards.

Self-Reflection and Ethical Awareness: This brain region is also involved in self-reflection and the understanding of ethical principles. Candidates must be able to assess their actions and intentions, ensuring they adhere to the core values of integrity and honor.

Temporal Lobes

Social Cognition and Empathy: The temporal lobes, particularly the superior temporal sulcus and the temporoparietal junction are involved in processing social information and empathy. For SFAS candidates, the ability to understand and consider the perspectives and emotions of others is vital for maintaining integrity in interactions and teamwork.

Memory and Learning from Past Experiences: The hippocampus, located in the temporal lobe, is key for memory formation. Candidates rely on memories of past experiences, including the outcomes of their actions and decisions, to guide future behavior in line with ethical standards.

Language and Communication Skills: Integrity also involves clear and honest communication, a function associated with the temporal lobes. For SFAS candidates, effectively communicating intentions, plans, and information truthfully is crucial.

Amygdala

Involved in emotional processing, influencing moral and ethical decisions.

- In selection, this area enables a candidate to make ethical decisions under stress and control one's emotions, demonstrating integrity in high-pressure, morally complex scenarios.

Integration in High-Stakes Environments

- Coordinated Functioning: The PFC, temporal lobes, and amygdala do not operate in isolation but rather work in tandem to support behaviors associated with integrity. The PFC's role in decision-making and impulse control, combined with the temporal lobes' involvement in social understanding and memory, forms the neural basis for integrity in SFAS candidates.
- Adaptability and Consistency: In the dynamic and challenging environment of SFAS, candidates must adapt

to rapidly changing situations while maintaining
consistent ethical standards. This adaptability is
supported by the integrated functioning of these brain
regions.

In summary, for an SFAS candidate, the prefrontal cortex and
temporal lobes are critical in fostering integrity. Their combined
functions enable candidates to make ethical decisions, control
impulses, understand the social and moral implications of their
actions, and communicate effectively and honestly, all of which are
essential for upholding the high standards of conduct expected in
Special Forces.

An in-depth understanding of how the amygdala, ventromedial
prefrontal cortex (vmPFC), and dorsolateral prefrontal cortex (dlPFC)
are interconnected and contribute to the trait of courage, particularly
in the context of an SFAS candidate.

Amygdala

Emotional Response and Fear Processing: The amygdala is a key
brain structure involved in processing emotions, especially fear. For
an SFAS candidate, facing high-risk, high-stress situations is
commonplace. The amygdala's response to perceived threats or challenging scenarios is crucial to experiencing and acknowledging fear,
an essential component of courage.

Threat Assessment: It evaluates potential threats and activates the
body's fear response. Recognizing and responding to danger effectively is vital for an SFAS candidate, who must often make quick,
high-stakes decisions.

Ventromedial Prefrontal Cortex (vmPFC)

Regulation of Emotional Responses: The vmPFC plays a crucial
role in regulating emotional responses, particularly those related to
fear generated by the amygdala. It helps modulate these responses,
enabling an SFAS candidate to remain calm and make rational decisions under pressure.

Risk Assessment and Decision-Making: This region is involved in
assessing risks and benefits, essential for making calculated decisions

in the face of danger. For an SFAS candidate, this means being able to evaluate the potential outcomes of actions realistically and choose the best course of action, balancing courage with caution.

Dorsolateral Prefrontal Cortex (dlPFC)

Executive Function and Cognitive Control: The dlPFC is key in executive functions, including planning, reasoning, and problem-solving. For an SFAS candidate, this involves strategizing, adapting plans on the fly, and solving complex problems, even amid stressful situations.

Overriding Automatic Fear Responses: The dlPFC helps override automatic fear responses. This capability is crucial for an SFAS candidate, who must often push beyond natural fear responses to achieve objectives and complete missions successfully.

Interplay in High-Stress Environments

- Balancing Fear and Action: The interplay between the amygdala, vmPFC, and dlPFC is essential for the manifestation of courage in an SFAS candidate. While the amygdala signals fear, the vmPFC and dlPFC work together to regulate this fear, enabling the candidate to face and overcome challenging situations.
- Integration for Courageous Behavior: These brain regions form a network that underlies the complex process of confronting fear and risks while maintaining the mental clarity to make strategic decisions and take calculated risks.

In summary, for an SFAS candidate, the amygdala's role in processing fear, combined with the vmPFC's function in emotion regulation and risk assessment, and the dlPFC's capacity for cognitive control, creates a neurological foundation for courage. This intricate neural interplay enables candidates to recognize and manage fear, assess and take calculated risks, and maintain decision-making capabilities under extreme stress, all of which are integral to demonstrating courage in the demanding realm of Special Forces selection.

In the challenging context of an SFAS candidate, the anterior cingulate cortex (ACC), the insular cortex, and the basal ganglia play significant roles in fostering the trait of perseverance. Let me elaborate on how these brain regions support the mental and emotional rigors faced by SFAS candidates.

Anterior Cingulate Cortex (ACC)

Error Detection and Conflict Resolution: The ACC is instrumental in monitoring actions and detecting errors or conflicts, especially during complex tasks. For an SFAS candidate, this means being able to quickly recognize and correct missteps or strategy errors during high-pressure tasks and assessments.

Pain Processing and Emotional Regulation: SFAS candidates undergo physically and mentally taxing challenges. The ACC is involved in processing physical pain and emotional distress. Its role in emotional regulation is crucial for candidates to manage stress, frustration, and fatigue, allowing them to continue pushing forward despite discomfort.

Motivation and Decision-Making: The ACC plays a role in the cognitive aspects of motivation, including the assessment of rewards and consequences. For an SFAS candidate, this involves evaluating the importance of their goals and the rewards of completing the selection process, which can help maintain motivation in the face of adversity.

Insular Cortex

Integrating emotional and cognitive processes: The insular cortex is involved in self-awareness, emotional regulation, and the perception of physical states, like pain and fatigue, and helps candidates assess their own physical and emotional state during stressful and demanding situations, contributing to their ability to persevere.

Interception and Bodily Awareness: The insular cortex is involved in interception, which is the perception of sensations from within the body. This internal awareness helps SFAS candidates understand and manage their physiological states (like stress or fatigue), enabling them to take responsibility for their health and well-being, which is vital in maintaining operational readiness.

Basal Ganglia

Habit Formation and Routine Execution: The basal ganglia are key in developing and executing routine behaviors and habits. During SFAS training, candidates perform numerous repetitive tasks and drills. The basal ganglia aid in forming these habits, making them more automatic and less mentally taxing over time.

Action Initiation and Perseverance in Tasks: These structures are crucial for initiating and sustaining actions. For an SFAS candidate, this means being able to start and persist in complex tasks, even when they are challenging, or the candidate is experiencing fatigue.

Reinforcement Learning and Behavior Modification: The basal ganglia are involved in learning from feedback and modifying behavior accordingly. This is essential for SFAS candidates as they adapt to the feedback received during training, fine-tuning their strategies and approaches for better performance.

Synergy in High-Stress Environments

- Resilience and Mental Toughness: The interaction between the ACC and basal ganglia is pivotal for developing resilience and mental toughness. The ACC's role in managing emotional responses and the basal ganglia's contribution to habit formation and action initiation create a neurological foundation for the perseverance required in SFAS.
- Adaptation and Learning: The capacity to adapt to new challenges, learn from mistakes, and modify behavior in response to feedback is a result of the dynamic interplay between these brain regions, essential for the rigorous demands of SFAS.

In summary, for an SFAS candidate, the coordinated functions of the ACC and basal ganglia are fundamental in supporting the high level of perseverance required. Their ability to manage stress, adapt to evolving challenges, and maintain motivation and focus is underpinned by these critical brain regions, contributing significantly to their success in such a demanding selection process.

The roles of the orbitofrontal cortex and the hippocampus concerning adaptability, especially within the challenging context of an SFAS candidate.

Orbitofrontal Cortex (OFC)

Decision-Making and Flexibility:

- The OFC is critically involved in decision-making processes, especially those requiring flexibility and adaptability. For an SFAS candidate, this involves making quick and often complex decisions in rapidly changing environments.
- The OFC helps in evaluating different options and outcomes, crucial for adapting strategies under uncertain and dynamic conditions.

Emotional Regulation and Social Behavior:

- The OFC also plays a role in emotional regulation and social behavior. An SFAS candidate needs to adapt not only to environmental changes but also to social dynamics within a team.
- The ability to read and respond appropriately to social cues, manage emotions, and navigate interpersonal relationships are all functions facilitated by the OFC, enhancing the candidate's adaptability in team-based scenarios.

Hippocampus

Memory Formation and Retrieval:

- The hippocampus is essential for the formation and retrieval of memories, particularly those involving spatial navigation and contextual information. For an SFAS candidate, remembering and utilizing past experiences and learned information is key to adapting effectively to new situations.

- The hippocampus allows candidates to apply lessons learned from previous training and experiences to new challenges, a fundamental aspect of adaptability.

Learning and Environmental Mapping:

- The hippocampus plays a role in spatial learning and environmental mapping. In the context of SFAS, candidates often navigate unfamiliar terrains and must quickly adapt to new geographic and situational contexts.
- The ability to form cognitive maps of new environments and recall spatial information is crucial for successful navigation and mission execution.

Interplay in Adaptability

- Decision-Making and Learning: The interaction between the OFC and the hippocampus is fundamental for adaptability. While the OFC contributes to flexible decision-making and emotional and social adaptation, the hippocampus supports this flexibility by providing contextual and experiential memory inputs.
- Dynamic Adaptation: For an SFAS candidate, this means being able to assess new situations rapidly, make informed decisions based on a combination of current contextual data and past experiences, and adjust emotional and social responses accordingly.

In summary, the orbitofrontal cortex and the hippocampus provide a neural basis for the adaptability required of an SFAS candidate. The OFC's involvement in flexible decision-making and emotional and social adaptation, combined with the hippocampus's role in memory and learning, equips candidates with the cognitive and emotional tools necessary to swiftly adjust to new challenges, environments, and team dynamics – all essential qualities for success in the demanding and unpredictable realm of Special Forces Assessment and Selection.

Let's elucidate how the prefrontal cortex and the insular cortex contribute to the concept of personal responsibility, particularly in the context of a Special Forces Assessment and Selection (SFAS) candidate.

Prefrontal Cortex (PFC)

Executive Functioning and Decision-Making: The PFC is central to executive functions, which include planning, decision-making, and impulse control. For an SFAS candidate, this means being able to make thoughtful decisions, plan ahead, and control impulsive actions, all of which are essential for taking personal responsibility in high-stakes situations.

Moral and Ethical Judgment: The PFC is involved in moral reasoning and ethical judgment. It allows SFAS candidates to evaluate the consequences of their actions not only for themselves but also for their team and the mission. This is crucial for taking responsibility for one's actions, especially in morally complex environments.

Self-Reflection and Awareness: This area of the brain also plays a role in self-awareness and reflection. An SFAS candidate must be able to assess their performance, acknowledge their strengths and weaknesses, and take responsibility for their personal development and actions.

Insular Cortex

Emotional Self-Awareness and Empathy: The insular cortex is key in processing and regulating emotions, as well as in developing empathy. For an SFAS candidate, being emotionally self-aware and empathetic is important for understanding the impact of one's actions on others, a fundamental aspect of personal responsibility.

Interception and Bodily Awareness: The insular cortex is involved in interception, which is the perception of sensations from within the body. This internal awareness helps SFAS candidates understand and manage their physiological states (like stress or fatigue), enabling them to take responsibility for their health and well-being, which is vital in maintaining operational readiness.

Integration of Emotional and Sensory Information: The insular cortex integrates emotional and sensory information, which is crucial for SFAS candidates to make balanced decisions that consider both logical and emotional aspects. This integration is essential for responsible decision-making in complex and often ambiguous situations.

Combined Role in Personal Responsibility

- Balanced Decision-Making: The PFC and insular cortex work together to enable SFAS candidates to make balanced decisions, considering both cognitive and emotional aspects, which is crucial for personal responsibility.
- - Self-Awareness and Adaptability: The combination of these brain areas supports self-awareness and adaptability. For an SFAS candidate, this means being aware of their own mental and physical states, understanding the impact of their actions, and being able to adapt behavior responsibly according to the demands of the situation.

In summary, the prefrontal cortex's role in executive functioning, moral judgment, and self-reflection, combined with the insular cortex's involvement in emotional awareness and bodily perception, form a neural basis for personal responsibility in SFAS candidates. These brain areas facilitate the ability to make responsible decisions, understand and manage one's emotions and physical states, and comprehend the wider impact of one's actions, all of which are essential for the high level of personal responsibility required in Special Forces training and operations.

Shedding light on how the prefrontal cortex and the temporal-parietal junction (TPJ) contribute to the trait of professionalism, particularly in the context of a Special Forces Assessment and Selection (SFAS) candidate.

Prefrontal Cortex (PFC)

Executive Functioning and Cognitive Control: The PFC is crucial for executive functions, which include planning, decision-making, and regulating behavior. For an SFAS candidate, these functions are essential for demonstrating professionalism, as they allow for organized, thoughtful, and strategic approaches to complex tasks and decision-making processes.

Social Behavior and Interaction: The PFC is involved in managing social interactions and behavior. It helps SFAS candidates navigate the nuances of professional military conduct, enabling them to act appropriately in a range of social and hierarchical contexts.

Moral and Ethical Reasoning: This brain region is also key in moral reasoning and ethical decision-making. Professionalism, especially in a military context, often involves ethical considerations, and the PFC plays a vital role in guiding candidates to make choices that align with professional and ethical standards.

Temporal-Parietal Junction (TPJ)

Social Cognition and Perspective-Taking: The TPJ is involved in social cognition, including the ability to understand and consider other people's perspectives, intentions, and beliefs. For an SFAS candidate, this is crucial in team-based activities and leadership roles, where understanding and respecting the viewpoints of others is a key aspect of professionalism.

Empathy and Understanding Others: The TPJ contributes to the capacity for empathy, which is the ability to understand and share the feelings of others. In a professional military environment, empathy enhances interpersonal relations and teamwork, both critical for SFAS candidates.

Theory of Mind: This area is also associated with the theory of mind, the ability to attribute mental states to oneself and others. For an SFAS candidate, this means being able to predict and understand the behavior of others, an important skill for professional interaction and collaboration.

Integration for Professionalism

- Holistic Functioning: The interaction between the PFC and TPJ is integral to the development and demonstration of professionalism. While the PFC aids in decision-making, ethical reasoning, and behavior regulation, the TPJ enhances social understanding and empathy.
- - Adaptability in Professional Contexts: For an SFAS candidate, these brain regions support the ability to adapt behaviors and decisions to professional military standards, understand and work effectively within a team, and maintain ethical standards even in high-pressure situations.

In summary, the prefrontal cortex and temporal-parietal junction collectively support the traits associated with professionalism in SFAS candidates. Their combined roles facilitate organized and ethical decision-making, appropriate social behavior, and empathy, enabling candidates to uphold high standards of professional conduct essential in Special Forces training and operations.

Elucidating how the motor cortex, cerebellum, prefrontal cortex, anterior cingulate cortex (ACC), and limbic system collectively contribute to the physical and mental capabilities essential for an SFAS candidate.

Motor Cortex

Movement Control and Coordination:

- The motor cortex is crucial for planning, controlling, and executing voluntary movements. For an SFAS candidate, this involves precise and coordinated physical actions, ranging from basic movements to complex tactical maneuvers.
- The fine-tuning of motor skills, essential for various physical aspects of SFAS training, is largely managed by this brain region.

Cerebellum
Balance and Motor Coordination:

- The cerebellum plays a key role in balance, coordination, and fine-tuning motor movements. Its function is vital for SFAS candidates who engage in physically demanding activities that require agility, balance, and precise motor control.
- It also assists in learning and mastering new physical skills, an ongoing requirement in SFAS training.

Prefrontal Cortex (PFC)
Cognitive Functioning and Decision-Making:

- The PFC is involved in executive functions such as planning, problem-solving, and decision-making. For SFAS candidates, this means the ability to strategize, make rapid decisions under stress, and adjust plans as needed.
- It also plays a role in attention and concentration, critical for both physical and mental tasks.

Anterior Cingulate Cortex (ACC)
Emotional Regulation and Pain Processing:

- The ACC is significant in regulating emotional responses and processing physical pain, essential for enduring the rigorous physical demands and stress of SFAS.
- It also contributes to motivational aspects, like perseverance and resilience, enabling candidates to push through physical and mental barriers.

Limbic System
Emotional Responses and Stress Management:

- The limbic system, which includes structures like the amygdala and hippocampus, is central to emotional processing and stress management.
- For an SFAS candidate, managing emotional responses and stress is crucial. The limbic system helps regulate emotions in high-pressure situations, maintaining mental stability.
- The hippocampus, part of the limbic system, is also involved in memory formation, important for learning and retaining tactical knowledge and skills.

Integrated Functioning for SFAS Candidates

- Coordinated Physical and Mental Performance: The motor cortex and cerebellum's roles in physical coordination and skill execution, combined with the PFC's, ACC's, and limbic system's contributions to cognitive processing, emotional regulation, and stress management, create a comprehensive network. This network is essential for the high-level physical and mental performance required of SFAS candidates.
- Adaptability and Resilience: The integration of these brain areas allows for adaptability and resilience, both physically and mentally. SFAS candidates must be able to quickly learn and master new skills, make decisions in complex and rapidly changing environments, and manage physical and emotional stress effectively.

In summary, the motor cortex, cerebellum, prefrontal cortex, anterior cingulate cortex, and limbic system collectively support the advanced physical and mental capabilities required for success in SFAS. Their interplay enables candidates to perform complex physical tasks, make strategic decisions, manage stress and emotional responses, and maintain motivation and resilience throughout the rigorous selection process.

Insights into how the prefrontal cortex, the temporal-parietal junction (TPJ), and the mirror neuron system contribute to the ability to be an effective team player, a critical trait for an SFAS candidate.

Prefrontal Cortex (PFC)

Decision-Making and Social Interaction:

- The PFC plays a significant role in decision-making and moderating social behavior. For an SFAS candidate, this involves making decisions that consider the welfare and dynamics of the entire team, not just individual success.
- It is also crucial for impulse control and adhering to social norms and rules, essential for maintaining harmony and effective collaboration within a team.

Cognitive Flexibility and Problem Solving:

- The ability to adapt thinking and approach to different situations (cognitive flexibility) and solve complex problems is rooted in the PFC. This flexibility is key for SFAS candidates in dynamic team environments where strategies and roles may rapidly change.

Temporal-Parietal Junction (TPJ)

Empathy and Perspective-Taking:

- The TPJ is involved in empathy and the ability to understand and consider the perspectives of others. Being empathetic and able to see from another team member's point of view is crucial for effective teamwork.
- This understanding aids in predicting and interpreting the actions and intentions of others, which is essential for coordination and cooperation in team-based tasks.

Social Cognition:

- The TPJ contributes to social cognition, which encompasses the ability to process and interpret social information. For an SFAS candidate, this means understanding complex social cues and responding appropriately in a team setting.

Mirror Neuron System
Imitation and Learning:

- The mirror neuron system is critical for the ability to observe and imitate the actions of others. In an SFAS setting, candidates often learn from and mimic the skills and tactics of their teammates and instructors.
- This system facilitates non-verbal learning and communication, which are vital for seamless team coordination and skill acquisition.

Empathy and Understanding Emotions:

- The mirror neuron system also plays a role in empathizing with others and understanding their emotions based on observed behaviors. This understanding fosters a cohesive team environment, which is essential in high-stress and collaborative missions.

Integrated Functioning in Team Dynamics

- Coordinated Teamwork: The integration of the PFC, TPJ, and mirror neuron system supports various aspects of being a team player. The PFC's role in decision-making and social regulation, combined with the TPJ's involvement in perspective-taking and social cognition, and the mirror neuron system's contribution to imitation and empathy, creates a comprehensive neural basis for effective teamwork.

- - Adaptability and Cohesion: These brain areas work together to allow an SFAS candidate to adapt to different team roles, understand and anticipate the needs and actions of other team members, and contribute positively to team dynamics and mission success.

In summary, the prefrontal cortex, temporal-parietal junction, and mirror neuron system collectively underpin the cognitive and empathetic skills necessary for being an effective team player. Their combined functions enable an SFAS candidate to make decisions considering team dynamics, understand and empathize with teammates, and learn from and synchronize with others, all of which are essential for successful collaboration in the demanding and interdependent context of Special Forces training and operations.

Conclusion: Integrating Neuroscience and Performance in Special Forces Training

Understanding the key qualities required for a Special Forces candidate, and having gained a reasonable understanding of the medical aspects related to these attributes, the question now arises: what are the next steps for someone aspiring to earn a Green Beret, even if they are not aiming to become a psychologist, neuroanatomist, academic professor, or a human performance expert? Individuals must be aware of their strengths and weaknesses to effectively allocate their time and effort in training, both physically and cognitively. Given the well-known benefits of physical exercise on brain function and health, and considering the intense physical preparation necessary for Special Forces selection, it's important to also focus on preparing mentally. Before arriving at Fort Bragg and Camp Mackall, what strategies can be employed to train the mental processes essential for maintaining focus, upholding core attributes, and managing mental health under challenging conditions such as cold, fatigue, hunger, injury, or pain? These situations are likely to occur, so having the mental resilience to confront them will be key to maintaining self-control amidst constant environmental stressors.

The core attributes necessary for a Green Beret include integrity, perseverance, capability, courage, personal responsibility, profession-alism, adaptability, and being a team player. Here are 20 examples of exercises and practices that can help train these attributes, keeping in mind the importance of balancing mental, cognitive, and physical training.

- **Endurance Training**: Long-distance running, rucking, and swimming build physical endurance and perseverance.
- **High-Intensity Interval Training (HIIT)**: Develops physical capability and mental toughness.
- **Team Sports**: Encourage teamwork and adaptability.
- **Martial Arts**: Enhances discipline, courage, and personal responsibility.
- **Rock Climbing**: Builds problem-solving skills and courage.
- **Yoga**: Improves flexibility, mindfulness, and stress management.
- **Meditation**: Enhances focus, mindfulness, and mental clarity.
- **Breathing Exercises**: Useful for stress management and relaxation.
- **Cold Exposure Training**: Builds mental toughness and adaptability.
- **Nutritional Planning**: Focuses on personal responsibility and professionalism in self-care.
- **Cognitive Games and Puzzles**: Enhance mental agility and problem-solving skills.
- **Language Learning**: Develops adaptability and cognitive flexibility.
- **Journaling**: Encourages reflection, integrity, and self-awareness.
- **Volunteering/Community Service**: Builds integrity and a sense of team spirit.

- **Visualization Practices:** Enhance mental preparation and focus.
- **Sleep Hygiene Practices:** Essential for cognitive function and physical recovery.
- **Direct Brain Stimulation Techniques (under expert guidance):** May enhance cognitive capabilities.
- **Time Management Exercises:** Develop personal responsibility and professionalism.
- **Stress Inoculation Training:** Prepares for high-pressure situations, enhancing courage and perseverance.
- **Outdoor Survival Skills Training:** Develops adaptability, problem-solving skills, and resilience.

The journey to elite performance in Special Forces is as much a cognitive endeavor as it is a physical one. The intricate tapestry of mental capabilities, attributes, and even the resilience that defines a Special Forces candidate, originates and is continuously orchestrated in the complex neural networks of the brain. These processes, often happening subconsciously, underscore the importance of understanding the neuroscientific underpinnings of our abilities.

Recognizing that physical prowess and mental fortitude are birthed in the same cerebral landscape is crucial. A fundamental level of knowledge about the physiology behind core attributes is indispensable for any candidate. This understanding enables individuals to accurately evaluate their strengths and weaknesses, discerning what aspects need sustaining and what requires improvement. It's a journey of self-awareness, powered by neuroscientific insights.

Although specific attributes are linked to distinct brain areas, it's imperative to understand that these are not siloed functions. Each region of the brain is a part of a larger, interconnected network, contributing to the fluid execution of complex tasks. This interconnectedness explains why cognitive training is as critical as physical training. The adage that 'the mind gives up before the body' holds a deep truth here. By comprehending the brain's role in performance, candidates can develop strategies to push beyond mental barriers, enhancing both individual and team performance.

This cognitive understanding is not just theoretical; it has practical applications in high-stress environments. Being able to conduct a self-evaluation in the heat of the moment, under duress, and an after-action review post-evolution, are skills that come from a deep understanding of one's neurological responses to stress and challenge. Learning from these moments is crucial for personal growth and for the improvement of the team.

The ultimate goal of understanding the neuroscience behind Special Forces preparation is not merely to pass the selection process. It's one of many components to be assessed by cadre to select individuals, with the right balance of physical strength and cognitive resilience. It's about preparing candidates not just to succeed but to excel in the roles expected of them. As we close, it becomes clear that the fusion of neuroscience and physical training is not just beneficial; it's essential for anyone aspiring to join the ranks of the most elite military units. This comprehensive approach is what sets apart a Special Forces candidate, preparing them not just to meet the challenges ahead but to redefine the limits of what is possible.

PROPERTY OF DR. SEAN BURKHARDT, Boulder FIT Health & Performance

BOTTOM LINE, it is essential to recognize that while physical prowess —comprising strength, endurance, flexibility, and precision in movement—is vital for the rigorous demands of selection, it is equally critical to cultivate optimal brain health and function. Your cognitive (decision-making) abilities, as much as your physical capabilities, are a direct reflection of your brain's functionality, which is indispensable for prospective Green Berets. The discussion of brain regions in this chapter is not intended to transform you into a neuroanatomist or psychologist but to underline the significance of these areas in fostering the cognitive processes essential for success in demanding roles. These neural networks operate tirelessly behind the scenes, supporting every action and decision, no matter the task at hand.

Our aim is to illuminate these critical areas and convey that they can be developed through targeted activities designed to stimulate neural pathways, leading to neuroplasticity, new synaptic connections, and enhanced brain function. The strategies presented are just the beginning; numerous other methods can be employed to effectively train these regions. During selection, you will face numerous challenges with unknown metrics amidst many variables. However, the one constant you can control is yourself. When you inevitably feel cold, hungry, and tired, you may doubt your ability to continue. Remember, your mental resilience, attitude, and determination often outweigh physical limitations and are crucial in controlling the continuous challenges you will face. If your brain functions effectively, it will help silence external distractions and focus your mind inward. This allows you to rely on your level of training rather than worrying about rising to the occasion.

Fact: These same brain regions not only influence but significantly enhance your physical performance for skills—hand-eye coordination, reaction time, tracking multiple objects simultaneously, and situational awareness. This deep-seated connection elevates your abilities in critical tasks, like shooting performance, far beyond what you initially perceive. It's not just necessary; it's transformative for all the cool guy shit. Recall the iconic scene from 1999 movie, *The Matrix*, where Morpheus leaps between buildings after urging Neo to "free your mind." While our goal is not to free your mind, we aim to educate you about the expectations and potential within you— empowering you to succeed. Let Neo free his mind. You, on the other hand, need to get selected and free the oppressed.

Cognitive Training Exercises

Nate has developed 80 Cognitive Training Exercises, divided into four categories:

- Self Awareness & Reflection

- Attention & Memory
- Critical & Creative Thinking
- Situational Awareness & Observation Skills.

We present them here as a master list so that you can review them for clarity, and we have already programmed them into your workouts. You will note that for nearly every ruck workout we have presented a Cognitive Prompt for you to engage in during your workout. We aim to achieve two functions with this programming. First, we want you to actually complete the prompt for the training value of the exercise. When we prompt you to "Reflect on the ARSOF attribute of 'Capability'" We want you to really do that. This is part of building self-awareness. These little exercises should prompt reflection and reconciliation. They should drive intellectual curiosity. Remember Nate's words, "Keep the meat-sack alive. Keep the meat-sack in some semblance of balance." If you can master this process of reflection *in* and *on* the moment, keep your brain engaged while under physical duress, and engage critically in the topic at hand then your ability to stay balanced will improve dramatically. Sure, you can hold up that heavy-ass apparatus, but can you also engage deliberately with your teammates and with assessing Cadre while doing so. Early in this process you might struggle to reflect *in* the moment and that's fine, but as the day closes out you should spend some time reflecting on the prompt and perhaps even journaling about it.

The second reason we are programming these in with the rucks is because every important decision that you make at SFAS you will make with a ruck on your back. If you go through your ruck prep with the bad habit of popping in your ear buds and blasting music to distract you from the process, then you are defeating yourself. You can't afford to be disconnected from the physical terrain around you, the human terrain that you are interacting with, or your body that is sending you valuable feedback. You can't afford this disassociation. We are programming you to specifically engage your brain when you put a ruck on. You'll be thankful for this default setting come Land Navigation Week.

An advanced technique might be to reconcile the prompt with one of the books from the reading list. If you can start to recognize related thoughts from separate disciplines, develop a practical connection, and put that connection into action then you are becoming formidable. The purpose of reading is to generate thinking. The purpose of writing is to organize our thinking. Don't just read. Read and think. Then read, think, write, and do.

Self-Awareness & Reflection

These exercises are designed to help you better understand yourself and the things that shape who you are, how you want to be, and your why. Without a clear knowledge of self, we are more likely to get derailed from our purpose or goal. Taking time to deliberately develop self-awareness is a trait of the highest performers. Reflection on ideas or concepts can help us to unlock new opportunities for growth.

- Reflect on the ARSOF attribute of 'Integrity'. Define it in your own words. Come up with ways you can demonstrate Integrity in action through the various known events of SFAS.
- Reflect on the ARSOF attribute of 'Courage'. Define it in your own words. Come up with ways you can demonstrate Courage in action through the various known events of SFAS.
- Reflect on the ARSOF attribute of 'Perseverance'. Define it in your own words. Come up with ways you can demonstrate Perseverance in action through the various known events of SFAS.
- Reflect on the ARSOF attribute of 'Personal Responsibility'. Define it in your own words. Come up with ways you can demonstrate a sense of Personal Responsibility in action through the various known events of SFAS.
- Reflect on the ARSOF attribute of 'Professionalism'. Define it in your own words. Come up with ways you can

demonstrate Professionalism in action through the various known events of SFAS.

- Reflect on the ARSOF attribute of 'Adaptability'. Define it in your own words. Come up with ways you can demonstrate Adaptability in action through the various known events of SFAS.
- Reflect on the ARSOF attribute of 'Team Player'. Define it in your own words. Come up with ways you can demonstrate being a Team Player in action through the various known events of SFAS.
- Reflect on the ARSOF attribute of 'Capability'. Define it in your own words. Come up with ways you can demonstrate your Capability in action through the various known events of SFAS.
- There are 5 SOF Truths. Reflect on each of these truths and come to terms with how the SFAS and SFQC process is designed to uphold these guiding principles.
- What are your top 3-5 strongest values? How do they align with the ARSOF attributes? Where there are differences, how can you leverage your personally held values to still embody the ARSOF values?
- Why are you going to SFAS? If you had to boil it down to 1 or 2 specific reasons, what would they be?
- What are your biggest strengths and qualities that you possess? Which new ones would you prioritize developing? How often do you allow yourself to lead with your strengths?
- If you could read the mind of the people closest to you, what would you hope their thoughts about you would look like?
- Reflect on what you are doing right now (i.e. running, rucking, etc.). How is this choice helping you get closer to your goals, but also move more in alignment to who you strive to be?

- What are examples from your life in which you failed to reach your expectations? What can you learn from those situations in order to make sure it doesn't happen this time around?
- Who is someone you look up to or hold as a role model? What are the characteristics that they have that inspire you?
- Reflect on the past week. What would you change? Where did you cut corners? What did you do well and need to continue doing?
- If you had a gun to your head and had to identify one moment in your life where you would do something differently, what would that one moment be? Why would you seek to change it, and what would you do?
- If (when) you achieve your goal of successful selection to Special forces, how would you change as a result? What would you DO differently from that point on? How would you act or feel differently?
- Explore any pain, unpleasantness, or discomfort you experience during this training day.What does this pain, and your willingness to experience it, tell you about what matters to you?How can this pain help you grow or develop? How can you learn from this pain?

Attention & Memory

These two cognitive functions go hand in hand. Attention is the foundation of all cognitive performance. If we can't develop stability of our mind and direct it to what's relevant, we fall victim to our circumstances rather than maintaining control over the reins. Retention of vital information is key to establishing a knowledge base, but you can't hope to remember what we haven't initial attended to in the first place. Train your attention in order to enhance your memory of both declarative and procedural knowledge.

- Reflect on the task of Land Navigation. What are the most common areas your attention gets directed to? Which things are relevant and relate to your effective execution of this task, and which things are merely 'noise' or distractors?
- Reflect on the Nasty Nick (or similar type obstacle course). What are the most common areas your attention gets directed to? Which things are relevant and relate to your effective execution of this task, and which things are merely 'noise' or distractors?
- Think about the swimming assessment. Regardless of your confidence level in swimming, where should you place your attention during this event? In your preparation for the event, where does your mind typically go? Does this help or hurt your performance?
- Reflect on team week. You will need to work collaboratively with other candidates, some of which you will not agree with or get along with. What are your triggers that typically interfere with your capacity to work well with others? What are the cues that allow you to ID them before they get in the way?
- You are doing some type of physical training right now. When you don't consciously direct your mind, where does it tend to wander off to? Begin to watch your mind and recognize when it starts to wander. When this happens, find something in your direct surroundings to bring you back to your main purpose for this session.
- Work to become simultaneously aware of your breathing pace as well as the terrain directly in front of you. Can you attend to both things? Is one easier than the other? What happens when one of these items dominates our attention?
- (For Rucking) What does the ruck feel like in my back? How are the straps positioned? How is the weight distribution? How does the weight of the ruck change

during each step or as I cover different terrain? How can this information help me refine how I prepare my ruck in the future?

- Commit this list of random items to memory. KIMS Game, List #1: 1. Candy Wrapper 2. Clay Pot 3. Keys 4. Rubber Duck 5. Piano 6. Spandex
- Commit this list of random items to memory. KIMS Game, List #2: 1. Lamp Shade 2. Cup 3. Radio 4. Camera 5. Sticky Note 6. Ice cube 7. Bottle
- Commit this list of random items to memory. KIMS Game, List #3: 1. Pool Cue 2. Controller 3. Cork 4. Needle 5. Ring 6. Toothpaste 7. Charger 8. Magnet
- Commit this list of random items to memory. KIMS Game, List #4: 1. Watch 2. Credit Card 3. Milk 4. Lotion 5. Tower 6. Pocket Knife 7. Wheel 8. Bolt 9. Sock
- Commit this list of random items to memory. KIMS Game, List #5: 1. Washing Machine 2. Sunglasses 3. Fence 4. Headphones 5. Bouquet 6. Shovel 7. Coat Hanger 8. Fork 9. Eyebrow 10. Shotgun
- Commit this portion of a standard packing list to memory. KIMS Game, List #6: 1. Duffel Bag 2. ID Tags 3. Patrol Cap 4. Blouse 5. Eye Protection 6. Running Shoes
- Commit this portion of a standard packing list to memory. KIMS Game, List #7: 1. Camelback Hydration System 2. Pen 3. Batteries 4. Razor 5. Shampoo 6. Deodorant 7. Headlamp
- Commit this list of military items to memory. KIMS Game, List #8: 1. Compass 2. Notebook 3. Canteen 4. Ammunition 5. Woobie 6. C-Wire 7. First-Aid Kit 8. NVGs
- Remember each of the primary missions of Special Forces: 1. Unconventional Warfare 2. Foreign Internal Defense 3. Special Reconnaissance 4. Direct Action 5. Combat Terrorism
- Remember this list of foreign languages that SF students may be required to learn: 1. French 2. Arabic 3. Chinese-

Mandarin 4. Persian-Farsi 5. Russian 6. Tagalog 7. Thai 8.
Levantine 9. Spanish

- Remember each phase of Unconventional Warfare & a
corresponding description: 1. Preparation 2. Initial Contact
3. Infiltration 4. Organization 5. Build Up 6. Employment 7.
Transition
- Remember each of the paragraphs of an OPORD & a
corresponding description: Situation, Mission, Execution,
Administration & Logistics, Command & Signal
- Remember each step of the Troop Leading Procedures in
order: 1. Receive the Mission 2. Issue Warning Order 3.
Make a Tentative Plan 4. Initiate Movement 5. Conduct
Reconnaissance 6. Complete the Plan 7. Issue Operation
Order 8. Supervise and Refine

<u>Critical & Creative Thinking</u>

As a Green Beret, you're expected to not only think deeply, but
think unconventionally. We must train this muscle, otherwise we will
default to our natural tendencies of instinct and intuition.
Summoning our capacity to exhibit mental effort is a skill, and one
you must be able to do when the situation arises. Creative thinking is
the manner in which we find options to solve complex problems. To
operate effectively in the gray area, you must be able to behave and
think flexibly.

- Solve this critical thinking question. What is one thing
that these items all have in common? job, polish, herb
(when first letter capitalized, you pronounce them
differently)
- Solve this critical thinking question. What is one thing
that these items all have in common? Jaguar, Falcon, Jet,
Bear, Charger (all of these are mascots for NFL teams)
- Solve this critical thinking question. Which is the odd
item out? Why? 2, 3, 5, 7, 11, 13, 17, 19, 23, 29, 33, 37 - 33 (All of
the rest are prime numbers)

- Solve this critical thinking question. Which is the odd item out? Why? (223x3), (3,345/5), (276+392), (6,021/9) - (276+392), all the other items =669

- Solve this critical thinking question. A man is looking at a photograph of someone. His friend asks who it is. The man replies, "Brothers and sisters, I have none. But that man's father is my father's son." Who was in the photograph? (His Son)

- Solve this critical thinking question. In 1990, a person is 15 years old. In 1995, that same person is 10 years old. How can this be? (The person was born in 2005 B.C.)

- Solve this critical thinking question. A bookworm eats a straight line through an encyclopedia consisting of ten parts sitting on a bookshelf. Each part has 1000 pages. The bookworm starts on the front cover of the first part and ends on the back cover of the last part. How many pages did the bookworm eat? (8000 pages)

- Solve this critical thinking, conditional logic question. Assume the following statement to be true: 'Whenever I go on a ruck march, I feel calm.' Which of the following variations of this statement are also true? A. 'If I feel calm, then I am on a ruck march.' (False) B. 'If I'm not on a ruck march, then I'm not feeling calm.' (False) C. 'If I'm not feeling calm, then I'm not on a ruck march.' (True)

- Solve this critical thinking, conditional logic question. Assume the following statement is true: 'I'll go to the bar, only if it's karaoke night.' Which of the following conditional structures this statement are also true? A. Karaoke night, therefore, I go to the bar (False) B. I go to the bar, therefore, it is karaoke night (True) C. I do not go to the bar, therefore, it is not karaoke night (False)

- Solve this critical thinking, flawed logic question. 'A comedy tour will be successful if it is well marketed and the comedian is established on social media. Evan is established on social media, and his tour was successful.

So his tour must have been well marketed.' Which of the following demonstrates a flawed line of reasoning that most closely resembles the flaw in logic in the above statement? A. This recipe will turn out only if one follows it exactly and uses high-quality ingredients. Arthur followed the recipe exactly and it turned out. Thus, Arthur must have used high-quality ingredients. (False) B. If a computer has the fastest microprocessor and the most memory available, it will meet Jordan's needs this year. This computer met Jordan's needs last year. So it must have had the fastest microprocessor and the most memory available last year. (False) C. If cacti are kept in the shade and watered more than twice weekly, they will die. This cactus was kept in the shade, and it is now dead. Therefore, it must have been watered more than twice weekly. (True) D. A house will suffer from dry rot and poor drainage only if it is built near a high water table. This house suffers from dry rot and has poor drainage. Thus, it must have been built near a high water table. (False) E. If one wears a suit that has double vents and narrow lapels, one will be fashionably dressed. The suit that Joseph wore to dinner last night had double vents and narrow lapels, so Joseph must have been fashionably dressed. (False)

- Complete this creativity exercise. Choose a random object. It can really be anything, such as a paper clip. Aim to generate as many possible uses for this object as you can.
- Complete this creativity exercise. Identify an object, word, thing, that you encounter. Come up with a story all about this particular item. The story can take whatever direction or turn that you want. There are no limits.
- Complete this creativity exercise. Choose a new idea or product that you've recently learned about. Go through the SCAMPER questions for that idea or product: Substitute: What can you trade from this idea for something else?Combine: What elements of this idea can

you combine for efficiency? Adapt: How can you adapt this idea for a different market? Modify: What can you modify to improve functionality? Put to another use: What's another use for this idea? Eliminate: What is unnecessary? Reverse: What can you adjust to make this project better?

- Complete this creativity exercise. Choose a new idea or product that you've recently learned about. Review the idea or product while 'wearing' each of the following thinking hats: Logic: The logic hat represents the facts related to the product or idea. Optimism: The optimism hat represents the possibilities for the product or idea with no barriers. Judgment: The judgment hat addresses the challenges or problems with the product or idea by considering the opposite point of view. Emotion: The emotion hat represents the feelings or perceptions associated with the project or idea. Creativity: The creativity hat introduces new ideas or possibilities for the idea or product. Management: The management hat oversees the discussion and makes sure the team represents all perspectives.
- Complete this creativity exercise. What is one problem that you continue to experience that you would love to solve? Identify and develop the concept of a tool that would allow you to solve this problem? What features would it include? What would this tool look like?
- Complete this creativity exercise. Select two random objects or items. Combine them into a new product. Develop a vision or strategy to 'sell' this new item to others. How would you convince them of the importance of this innovative item? What things would you attempt to appeal to in order to get them bought in?
- Complete this creativity exercise. Develop a 6-word story. Once you've created the story, allow yourself to think about the details of the story. Fill in the gaps. Repeat this

as many times as necessary until you've completed your
training session for the day.

- Complete this creativity exercise. Attempt to think in a
  way that eliminates the words: "I", "Me", "My", and "Mine".
  Broaden the way in which you interact with your mind
  and the dialogue it generates.
- Complete this creativity exercise. Pick someone in your
  life who you deeply care about. Attempt to put yourself in
  his or her shoes. How do they feel about your preparation
  for SFAS? What does it look like from their perspective?
  Do they understand why you are striving towards this
  goal? How do they view your actions and choices?
- Complete this creativity exercise. Come with a new
  thought, idea, observation, etc. every minute on the
  minute. There are no rules or parameters around what
  you come up with. The goal is just to generate something
  new each minute of your training session.

Situational Awareness & Observation Skills

Your performance ultimately happens in whatever environment
you find yourself. This environment, especially in Special Operations, is dynamic. This requires us to constantly update our situational awareness in order to respond to changes as they occur. Every
second counts in a fire fight or even during a Key Leader Engagement. We can enhance the detail we pick up from our environments
through training the skill of observation. Once again, however, this is
something you must be intentional about training.

- Become aware of your surroundings. Have you run/rucked
  in this gym/trail/road before? Whether or not you have,
  reflect on what things in this environment that you have
  either seen before or are familiar to things you have seen
  before. What things are unique or novel to your PT today?
- Today you will be prioritizing the different things that
  you hear in your surroundings. See if you can identify all

the various sounds around you. When you identify a
sound, allow yourself to label or categorize it, and then
broaden your awareness back out to look for more. Try
not to get 'stuck' thinking or wondering about any
particular sound.

- Focus on how you are changing the environment around
you. How much noise or sound is being generated by you
alone? What evidence of your presence is left behind in
this space? Are you disturbing, in any way, the natural
manner of things? Can you minimize your impact by
becoming consciously aware of it?

- Maintain a soft focus on a short distance in front of you.
As you move in the environment, recognize how the visual
scene changes, but do so in a way that maintains this soft
focus. When your eye sharpens around specific details or
features, acknowledge it but bring it back to that soft
focus.

- Identify the fluctuations of the ground or surface you are
moving upon. How do changes in your weight distribution
or balance inform you about the terrain? As your body
moves, it is directly interacting with the greater
environment. Each subtle movement, and your
proprioceptive awareness, feed information to you. Study
your body as it moves through space. This is especially
important when moving under load.

- What information can you gather using your sense of
smell? What do you smell and how does it change over
time? Whenever these sensations retreat to the
background, consciously become aware of the things that
you smell.

- Allow your mind to get lost on something in your
surroundings. Find something that interests you, it can be
anything at all. Generate questions about that thing, study
it and pick out details about it. See how long your mind
will linger on that feature of your environment until it is

ready to find something new. Repeat this with different objects around you until your PT is complete.

- Study any other people who you encounter today during your workout. As you pass them or see them, make a point to focus on their facial features (clothing, height, eight, etc.). What are the things that stand out to you? What inferences might you make about this person? Would you be able to pick them out in a crowd if you saw them again?
- Feel the temperature of your environment. Are you: hot, warm, comfortable, cool, cold, etc.? What sensations make you more aware of the temperature and how it affects you? Do you notice the temperature of the air as you breathe in/out? Is there a breeze or fan blowing on your skin? Is your choice of clothing appropriate for maintain your current level of comfort?
- Set your attention on the external environment around you. Each time your attention gets distracted or pulled away by something internal (i.e. a thought, sensation, memory, emotion, etc.), take note of it and re-direct to something nearby. As this continues to happen, try and place a simple label on that experience that is pulling you out of the present moment.
- Train the shift between situational awareness and self-awareness. Imagine three general levels for your mind to attune to: your breath, your body, your external environment. Intentionally shift your attention between each of these 3 specific stages of knowing. Focus on the breath. Shift to focusing on your body with a complete body scan. Shift to the world around you. Repeat this process, aiming to make each shift as efficient as possible.
- Observe your surroundings as if you were a cartographer. Observe the changes in elevations and the landmarks in your environment. What would these look like if you were reading a map? Visualize it clearly in your mind's eye.

- Observe your surroundings as if you were prepping an ambush or raid. What are the features of the environment you could use to your advantage? What are the potential pitfalls of using this space? Do this exercise every ~400 meters as the terrain changes.
- What are the primary forms of vegetation in this area? Can you spot different types of trees? What are the specific features of each type of vegetation that stand out to you? As you observe the plant life in your surroundings, what other features of your environment become more noticeable to you? How could you leverage this during different military tasks?
- Allow your mind to get lost on something in your surroundings. Find something that interests you, it can be anything at all. Generate questions about that thing, study it and pick out details about it. See how long your mind will linger on that feature of your environment until it is ready to find something new. Repeat this with different objects around you until your PT is complete.
- Study any other people who you encounter today during your workout. As you pass them or see them, make a point to focus on their facial features (clothing, height, eight, etc.). What are the things that stand out to you? What inferences might you make about this person? Would you be able to pick them out in a crowd if you saw them again?
- Today, use a device (preferably a cell phone) to recognize how much information we miss from our surroundings when we get sucked into technology. Scroll through your phone, change the song you are listening to, review heart rate data, ready something, etc. Make a point to intentionally busy yourself on your phone. At the end of the workout, reflect on how that experience differed from the workouts in which you gainfully employed your mind on details of the experience itself. Which did you prefer?

Why? What are the potential drawbacks of each
approach?

- Seeing what is missing can sometimes be as important as
  seeing what is there. As you navigate your surroundings,
  reflect on what is not present to your eye that you find
  surprising or interesting. As you identify potential things
  that are missing, question why that may be the case.
- See to remember. Pay particular attention to the route and
  direction you travel. What are the twists, turns, and bends
  in the path that you took or chose not to take? When you
  complete you exercise for the day, take a notebook page
  and see how detailed you can re-create this path and some
  of the things that occurred to you at key landmarks.
- Observe your observation tendencies. This is a very 'meta'
  exercise, however it is important to identify our go-to
  tendencies to better understand our potential limitations.
  When you aim to observe or pick up details from your
  environment, what are your typical steps in the process?
  How can intentionally choosing a different starting point
  for observation help you to see even more?

8

SKILLS

We treat the body rigorously so that it will not be disobedient to the mind.
- Seneca

You need to be useful, to both you and others. So we need to build skills. Some of these skills are tactile *hard skills*, like tying knots. Some of these skills are *soft skills*, like communication. Some of them are physical in nature, like balance. And others are cerebral, like effective listening. So hard and soft and physical and cerebral, skills are important. And they are rarely inherent. You might have naturally good balance, but they are definitely qualities that you can train. We are going to train them. Some of this training will be stand-alone efforts. We will dedicate some *skills only* sessions, but really these are just intentional rest days that we don't want to waste. But much of the skills training is integral to other workouts. Interconnected.

Deciding which skills are the most critical is no small task, because all the rules matter, and you must train everything. Most coaches agree on the Big 6 - agility, balance, coordination (hand-eye and/or foot/eye), power, reaction time, and speed. We agree, but we think that you need less descriptive and more prescriptive, so we are adding to this list. Take balance for example. Walking a balance beam is certainly training an athletic skill and one that you might see on the Nasty Nick obstacle course. But what about walking on a downed tree with a ruck on your back, after walking for 10 miles, at night? It's still balance, but it's that unique SFAS environment that we need to account for. An uneven and unstable log, likely a little wet, in the middle of a draw, crossing a creek, a 75-pound ruck pressing on your traps, your legs are smoked, and you are convinced that you hear banjo music in the distance. Is that still balance, but significantly different than a balance beam? If your program was developed by a guy who doesn't understand SFAS then how can the program account for this unique training environment?

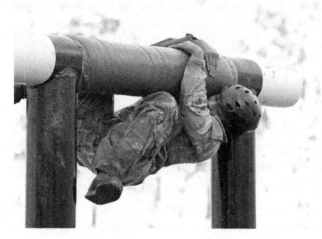

Have You Practiced This Skill?

Now were not advocating for building a replica of *The Tough One* in your backyard. And we definitely aren't suggesting that you when you get on the treadmill that you carry an E-Z Curl bar to replicate a weapon. But that critical *field-based* component that is so central to our ruck programming should make some appearances. If you have access to an obstacle course, then use it!

Listed below is a menu that we have selected. Much like the mobility menu you have a role to play here. You must determine what skills you are lacking and choose from the menu to address them. Your skills workout should change over time as you develop some skills and others atrophy. A constant reflection on your performance is important. It may take a few sessions to get a good flow figured out. You might never get great at a particular skill; you should keep working on that one. You might master a skill quickly; you should focus on other skills so that you can master them.

Skills List

1. Knot Tying – rope, tubular nylon
2. Rope Climbing
3. Mantling
4. Balance – loaded, unloaded, asymmetrically loaded, at height
5. Handstands
6. Comfort with heights
7. Comfort with enclosed spaces
8. Underhand Ball Catch – small, large, weighted
9. Underhand Ball Throw – small, large, weighted
10. Overhand Throw – small, large, weighted
11. Overhand Catch – small, large, weighted
12. Juggling - hand-eye coordination
13. Explosive Jumping – loaded, unloaded
14. Dynamic Landing – loaded, unloaded
15. Falling – forward, backwards, side
16. Bike Riding
17. Swimming
18. Tree Climbing
19. Turkish Get Up
20. Pistol Squats
21. Footwork – Agility Ladder - forward, backwards , lateral
22. Hopping - forward, backwards , lateral
23. Turning - loaded, unloaded
24. Sprawling - loaded, unloaded
25. Jumping rope -forward, backwards , lateral
26. Dribbling - forward, backwards , lateral
27. Cone Weave - forward, backwards , lateral
28. Hurdles, mini hurdles - forward, backwards , lateral
29. Shuffle runs - forward, backwards , lateral
30. Pit Stop – How fast can you change socks on a ruck workout

9

HOW TO USE THIS PERFORMANCE JOURNAL

A problem written down is a problem halved. -Kidlin's Law

There is a method to this particular madness of *Shut Up and Ruck* SFAS prep. We have very carefully programmed each day to give you just the right amount of stimulus. We are covering, very deliberately, all six pillars of Operational Fitness. We are preparing for the most demanding assessment environment that you could imagine, so this process is comprehensive to the extreme. You are working as hard as possible, but you are resting with just as much deliberate effort. We are fueling this endeavor with clean, high-quality food. We are preparing our minds to both *reflect **on the moment***, so that we can grow as a human and we are learning to *reflect **in the moment*** so that we don't miss opportunities to be correctly assessed.

Reflection

This is the purpose of this journal methodology. Reflection. I have repeatedly noted that SFAS isn't just about Selection, it's more about

Assessment. The Cadre are going to watch everything that you do, everything that you present about yourself, and render a judgement of your behavior and performance. If you don't understand *how* you present yourself, you won't be able to properly broadcast yourself. The Cadre shall think of you what you allow them to think of you. And you will not have unlimited opportunities to get things "just right" for those opportunities. As such, you need to take advantage of every opportunity that you get. You must learn to reflect *in* the moment. This differs from reflecting *on* the moment, in that reflecting *on* the moment is something that you do after the fact. Once the task is complete you often sit and think, "How did I do? What could I have done better? How were my actions perceived?" Have you ever replayed an argument in your head and thought, "Oh! I wish I had said this instead"; that is reflecting *on* the moment. And while that is very valuable and will certainly dominate your reflection activity early on in this process, it is less valuable than also being able to reflect *in* the moment.

Reflecting *in* the moment is the ability to recognize your behavior *while* it is happening so that you can then modify that behavior, so it is reflective of both your true self and presents the best possible assessment opportunity. This is self-awareness. Remember, the Cadre shall think of you what you allow them to think. If you can deliberately manage how you present yourself, then you should do so. Reflecting *in* the moment enables you to do so. I have often seen Candidates who were unable to recognize, *in* the moment, just how poorly they were behaving early in the day or early in the iteration of an event. The Cadre make note of that and that anchors their perception of that Candidate the rest of the day. And it goes the other direction as well. If you can perform well, and recognize it *in* the moment, and note how that impacts the situation (situational awareness) then you can start to manipulate the situation to your advantage. But it's cumulative. You can't manipulate the situation if you are not aware of the situation, and you can't be aware of the situation if you are not aware of yourself. So learning who you are is foundational to this process. This is reflection.

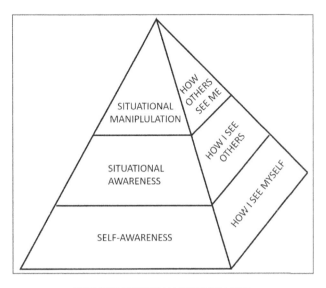

THE HUMAN DYNAMICS PYRAMID

We have raised an entire generation of potential candidates that have been exposed to a lack-luster curated self-awareness environment. Authority figures are feeble and mute. Traditional two parent households are becoming less common, so our young men (and women) are losing this invaluable masculine feedback mechanism. Youth participation in team sports is precipitously low and dropping. And the sports most impacted are tackle football, lacrosse, and wrestling: traditional, full-contact, in-your-face, resilience building sports (Institute, 2023). And ones that require a coach. A coach that tells you exactly how you are performing and requires you to acknowledge it. So many young men lack this critical foundational step of self-awareness. This journaling process seeks to address this. You're not just writing this stuff down for the sake of writing it down. Write it down, read it, review it, and make sense of it. This is who you are.

Analog vs Digital

There is a reason why we are deliberately making this a largely analog effort. Analog is superior to digital in recall and comprehension (Umejima, Ibaraki, Yamazaki, & Sakai, 2021) (Askvik, Weel, &

Meer, 2020) (Singer & Alexander, 2016). There are some great apps that can help you and we've already extolled the virtues of digital remote coaching. But analog is superior. So this program is old school, pen and paper, write it down, and re-read it. More anti-marketing. A login and password and a flashy app is easy enough to produce. That's why there are so many out there. We want this to be tactile. Write down what you do, then read what you write. Go back over your performance every week. Then every month. Take note of patterns and trends. Adjust your mobility and warmup routines to adapt this program to your specific weaknesses. In other words, coach yourself and let this journal be the adjudicator of your performance. The data does not lie.

The Importance of Habit

You're not going to wake up Monday morning and be perfect and put together a flawless string of impeccable days. You're not going to make a plan on Sunday that survives perfectly all the way through Saturday. It's just not going to happen. Life happens. Shit happens. Be prepared for enemy contact. If you miss a day, then pick it back up the next. Keep making plays. If you miss a week, then do that week again. Don't just keep going because the time is ticking. The time will always tick, you must perform. If your ruck time sucked, then get into your data and figure out if it's something that you can change. Maybe it's just a bad day. Maybe it's because you're sleeping and eating like an amateur. But you won't know this unless you write everything down and are diligent in reviewing your performance. You are building self-awareness and you are identifying where you can improve. And it takes time.

Here is the amazing part about habit. First, it helps you to codify beneficial behavior. You know, especially after reading the first 8+ chapters, exactly what you need to do. You know what you need to eat and drink. You know that you're not supposed to stay up late doomscrolling on your phone. You know that you're supposed to work on your mobility and skills. You know exactly what you need to do and if you forgot? Well, all you have to do is open each page and follow that day's instructions. If you are deliberate about doing the little things that we are already telling you to do, the big things, like performance gains, will come. It just takes time. The second great thing about habit and routine is that humans thrive in that environment (Arlinghaus & Johnston, 2019). This program, this process, and this journal are all seeking to take all of the guess work out of your SFAS prep. You will make routine the type of behavior that produces results. All you have to do is follow the program. Get in the habit of high performance.

The Three Phases

This program follows three phases. The first two months are the base building phase. Learn to lift, learn to run, focus on form, and start to gain mobility and flexibility. You will build the cardio capacity that will help you run and ruck faster. But first, you will run slowly. Let your body work the way that it is designed to work. Let physiological adaptations occur. And start to learn skills. Learn to climb a rope. Learn balance. Learn to control your body. You are building a foundation here, so build it well. Later, in the next phases, you will build the brick house. This foundation is performance based, not time. Once you can bench press .85 x your bodyweight, squat 1 x your bodyweight, deadlift 1.5 x your bodyweight, and run continuously (unbroken) for 90 minutes at Zone 2 and only once you can meet all of these benchmarks you can move to the next phase. If you can already meet these performance benchmarks, and your mobility, flexibility, and skills are appropriately supportive then you can move to the next phase. You will start the reading list. Pick a book and read it. Take notes. Teach yourself. Be a man of impact and significance. Graphic novels are comic books. Comic books are for kids. Men read books and make sense of the ideas. Follow the mental cues that we present you. You're not just working out, you're becoming formidable.

The second phase is the capacity building phase. You have laid the proper foundation and now the true construction begins. You have readied your joints and you have established the proper neural pathways. The pump is primed, and it is time to fill the tank. And perhaps most importantly, it is time to start rucking. That's right, there is no rucking except for a single diagnostic in phase one. But now we have built the prerequisite strength and cardio baseline, and we can begin rucking. Slowly and with light weights, at first, but we will soon be up to speed as we ready ourselves for the 5x5 Man Maker. You'll start to really toughen your feet and build resilience. We'll also start introducing some cognitive load during your physical preparedness. You'll tie knots during a ruck to train fine motor skills during gross motor activities. You'll work memory recall when your brain is already taxed. And you'll really learn how to dial in your recovery, sleep, and nutrition efforts. You will start to note how much your performance suffers when you disregard these critical elements. That data doesn't lie. You will keep reading. But now you're also a writer. You just spent a few months writing down everything that you consume and do. So you're a writer.

Again your advancement in the program is performance based, not time. Once you can demonstrate the requisite strength – bench press 1 x bodyweight, squat 1.5 x bodyweight, and deadlift 2 x bodyweight as well as maintain 90 minutes continuous running at Zone 2, then you can move to the next phase. And your rucking in this phase is about understanding technique. Learn to shuffle and understand how to pace. Learn to manipulate the load, adjust your straps, and manage the misery. You are now ready for the finishing phase. If you are ahead of your desired timeline, then it is in this phase that you should drift. The final few months are intense and loitering in that zone could put you at risk. This task seems daunting now, but at the four-month mark of this program you will have a much better sense of your response to stimuli because you will be keeping good notes and building good habits and routines.

The third and final phase is where we put this all together. Your lifting will be just something that you do. It's a habit now. You will be putting in intense workouts, strengthening your grip beyond measure, and examining any lagging performance and addressing these shortcomings. Are your pushups lagging? You will develop an enhanced pre-mobility/warm-up routine to work on this. Are your runs lagging a bit? You will adjust the *2-3 times a week* format to incorporate a speed session in lieu of the third 5x5. You are mastering your prep and nothing gets forgotten. You will be well read. You will have a better vocabulary. You will be able to tell stories and are a good listener. You are an effective communicator. You are resilient. You are formidable. You are worthy of being Selected.

What To Do - The Data Does Not Lie

The first week is all assessments. Some things you will do well. Some things you will do poorly. Sometimes you won't be able to do the things. This is a starting position. This is part of the process. This is how you start to build self-awareness. *The data does not lie.* It is what it is. So just do the assessments as they are laid out. Write down how you did. Move on to the next event. At the end of the week, you will assess how you did. You will review the data and determine where you need work. If you did 10 HRPUs, then your warm-up/mobility/pre-hab will now include some HRPU sets. If your FMS revealed poor shoulder mobility, then you will address this deficiency. If your 1 Rep Max is surprisingly weak (we don't care what you used to lift, we care what are lifting right now) then your diet is going to include excess calories to fuel some significant muscle growth. You are following the program as we laid it out, but this is not something that is just happening *to* you. This is something that is happening *through* you. You have agency of elements of this process. The warm-up/mobility/pre-hab routine in particular, but also the performance nutrition, sleep hygiene, reading list, and skills work. Yes, trust the process AND do your part in the process. We have provided an excellent menu, your job is to execute with intensity, intention, and purpose.

Follow the prompts and track everything. You are a mad scientist, and your performance is the ultimate experiment. Remember system thinking and test your response to different inputs. Only change one thing in one domain at a time, otherwise you won't be able to isolate the variables, but you are in charge of your progress. So, be in charge. At the end of each phase you will take another assessment. If you pass the assessment, then you advance to the next phase. If you don't pass the assessment, then you have to repeat the last week until you can pass. *The data does not lie.* Go to the Performance Journal and look at what a perfect week looks like.

Aim to finish the program a week or two prior to reporting to SFAS. You don't necessarily need a deload time, but you want to be ready and rested. It's a difficult balance but nobody will be able provide better feedback than you. You are in charge. You are ready.

WHEN DO I NEED A COACH?

This program, this book, and this entire process is specifically designed to work without a coach. You are essentially self-coaching. But I have come to respect, a great deal, the value of good coaching. Seventy percent of aspiring candidates likely won't need additional coaching. Thousands of operators have gone before you without the benefit of even a decent program, so actual professional coaching seems almost decadent. Paying someone to coach seems nearly obscene. But I often find that those that think they don't need coaching are usually the most in need of it. Conversely, those that recognize the value of good coaching often require the least amount of it.

And I should note that most coaching isn't some deep, committed, long term relationship. It certainly can be. But sometimes you just need a little tweak or a small boost. And a very little intervention early on in a process can help you set good patterns and habits that have an exponential return on investment. A quick consult when you identify a potential issue can keep your performance from ever suffering. Sometimes you just need someone to tell you shut up and work. You probably know what you need to do, but having someone else tell you is more impactful.

So here is my broad guidance on coaching. As you start this program you will be collecting a ton of data. If you are struggling to make sense of this data or turn it into improved performance, then you probably need a coach. If you are lagging in a particular domain inconsistently with your other improvements, then you probably need a coach. If you have a nagging injury that just won't go away, then you probably need a coach. If you just can't seem to master a particular movement no matter how hard you try, then you probably need a coach. And if you are perpetually struggling to meet the performance benchmarks or otherwise hold yourself to the schedule, then you probably need a coach. Some guys just need a little accountability forcing function.

Dave, Sean, Halley, and Nate are my go-to coaches, and you already see how good they are. I suspect that they will quickly have a client list that exceeds their capacity, but if you can secure a coveted spot on their roster then I would strongly encourage it. But there are hundreds of amazing professionals that we couldn't include in our printed endorsement. As this goes to print, we already have a network of several dozen across the United States. Some coaches don't believe in the exact program we developed; they are still great coaches. SFAS is different, so *our* coaches need to be as well. Many more coaches will emerge as they discover our program. We intend to maintain a roster of like-minded professionals on our website, TFVooDoo.com. There is no franchise fee or certification or business model. We are not gatekeepers, we are guides. If you need coaching, check our website. If you are a coach and you want to be included in our network, then send us a note. There are no fees, and the only price of admission is that you share our philosophy:

- Simple, not easy.
- All the rules matter, all the time.
- The data doesn't lie
- Basics build champions.
- Faster than the strongest lifter, stronger than the fastest runner.

- PC, not beret.
- Good men will not just sit and watch other men suffer.

IF YOU WANT to work with Coach David Hsu then send him a message at davidhsucoaching@gmail.com.

If you want to work with Dr. Sean Burkhardt or Halley Burkhardt then you can reach them via their website, neurostrongcolorado.com or at alpharesolutegroup.com.

If you want to work with Mr. Nate Toft then you can contact him via topdogdevelopmentconsulting.com.

READING LIST

The purpose of knowledge is action, not knowledge. -Aristotle

Here it is, my reading list. I have resisted creating a reading list, but I must give the people what they want. The *people* are *relentless.* I spent no small amount of time curating this list and I'm still not certain that its definitive, but it's a great start. I have broken this into four categories; SF Baseline, Psychology and Human Nature, History, and Performance. The SF Baseline stuff is what I consider to be the seminal texts. There are certainly many more excellent books, but these give you a good idea of the more recent history of the Regiment while also being well written stories. Psychology is a vast field and I make no representation that this list is exhaustive. That's why they make you go to college to get credentialed, but this list will give you a practitioner's guide to psychology and human nature. I have avoided too much of the Ancients as authors in favor of insightful history of the Ancients. It's just easier to read and more helpful. You might prioritize reading the human performance stuff up front in this process.

They will help shape your understanding of the deeply complex topic and might even help you when you craft your mobility and warm-up routines.

I recommend getting these books in physical print (analog is superior to digital). You should have a library. Drunkards have man caves; formidable men have libraries. Even better if your library has a bar in it. You may note that there is no popular fiction on this list. I read every single day and admittedly the bulk of my reading is popular fiction. But I do this type of reading as part of my sleep routine, and I would struggle to recall much. It's mostly vapid trash and it's always digital. But my real physical library is mine. I reference it often and I have read every single one of these books, many of them multiple times. So build your library and start it with these books.

Special Forces Baseline

1. *Ruck Up or Shut Up: The Comprehensive Guide to Special Forces Assessment and Selection* – David Walton
2. *Masters of Chaos: The Secret History of Special Forces* - Linda Robinson
3. *Five Years to Freedom: The True Story of a Vietnam POW* - James N. Rowe
4. *Hammerhead Six: How Green Berets Waged an Unconventional War Against the Taliban to Win in Afghanistan's Deadly Pech Valley* - Ronald Fry and Tad Tuleja
5. *The Guerrilla Factory: The Making of Special Forces Officers, the Green Berets* - Tony Schwalm
6. *The Only Thing Worth Dying For: How Eleven Green Berets Forged a New Afghanistan* - Eric Blehm
7. *The Ugly American* - Eugene Burdick and William Lederer

Psychology/Human Nature

1. *12 Rules for Life: An Antidote to Chaos* - Jordan Peterson
2. *How To Win Friends and Influence People* - Dale Carnegie

3. *Atomic Habits: An Easy & Proven Way to Build Good Habits & Break Bad Ones* - James Clear
4. *Thinking, Fast and Slow* - Daniel Kahneman
5. *Man's Search For Meaning* - Viktor Frankl
6. *Willpower: Rediscovering the Greatest Human Strength* - Roy Baumeister
7. *Read People like a Book: How to Analyze, Understand, and Predict People's Emotions, Thoughts, Intentions, and Behaviors: How to Be More Likable and Charismatic* - Patrick King
8. *48 Laws of Power* -Robert Greene
9. *The Bible – A man who only has faith in himself has no faith at all.*

History

1. *From Cyrus to Alexander: A History of the Persian Empire* - Pierre Briant
2. *All the Shah's Men: An American Coup and the Roots of Middle East Terror* – Stephen Kinzer
3. *The War Before the War: Fugitive Slaves and the Struggle for America's Soul from the Revolution to the Civil War* – Andrew Delblanco
4. *Powers and Thrones: A New History of the Middle Ages* – Dan Jones
5. *Conquistador: Hernan Cortes, King Montezuma, and the Last Stand of the Aztecs* - Buddy Levy
6. *1491: New Revelations of the Americas Before Columbus* - Charles Mann
7. *Children of Ash and Elm: A History of the Vikings* - Neil Price
8. *SPQR: A History of Ancient Rome* - Mary Beard
9. *Rubicon: The Last Years of the Roman Republic* - Tom Holland
10. *Dynasty: The Rise and Fall of the House of Caesar* - Tom Holland

11. *The Anglo-Saxons: A History of the Beginnings of England* - Marc Morris
12. *The Plantagenets: The Warrior Kings and Queens Who Made England* - Daniel Jones
13. *Ancient Greece - Creators, Conquerors, and Citizens* - Robin Waterfield
14. *The Rise and Fall of Ancient Egypt* - Toby Wilkinson
15. *Genghis Khan and the Making of the Modern World* - Jack Weatherford
16. *Persian Fire: The First World Empire and the Battle for the West* - Tom Holland
17. *Rome and Persia: The Seven Hundred Year Rivalry* - Adrian Goldsworthy

Performance

1. *Sleep Smarter: 21 Essential Strategies to Sleep Your Way to A Better Body, Better Health, and Bigger Success* - Shawn Stevenson
2. *Eat It!: The Most Sustainable Diet and Workout Ever Made: Burn Fat, Get Strong, and Enjoy Your Favorite Foods Guilt Free* - Jordan Syatt and Mike Vacanti
3. *Human Performance for Tactical Athletes* - o2x Human Performance
4. *Daniels Running Formula* - Jack Daniels
5. *Becoming a Supple Leopard* - Dr. Kelly Starrett

THE BEST WAY

- The best way to build strength is *to follow the principle of progressive overload, usually with intense weightlifting, focused on compound movements.*
- The best way to build rucking performance is *field based progressive load carriage, usually 2-3 times a week, focused on short intense sessions.*
- The best way to fuel performance is *balanced whole foods, usually unprocessed, focused on proper protein intake.*

THE 5X5 - THE MAN MAKER

The 5x5 is the culmination for THE BEST methodology to improve rucking performance. The best way to improve rucking performance is field based progressive load carriage, usually 2-3 times a week, focused on short intense sessions.

Start with building the prerequisite strength of .85 x BW bench press and 1.25 x BW squat. Simultaneously work on building aerobic base with Zone 2 running for 90 minutes unbroken. Once you can do this, you can start rucking.

Build slowly in both distance and weight. Maybe start with 2 miles rucking at 20 pounds and 20 minutes running. As you adapt, slowly increase weight, distance, and pace until you get to 5 miles rucking at 12-13 minute miles @55 pounds and 5 miles running at 7 minute miles.

The entire session should be completed within 2 hours; 90 minutes is competitive. You should change into running shoes for the run portion, but rucking in PT clothes violates the 3 rules.

The 5x5 - The Man Maker

5 mile ruck

100 squats with ruck

5 mile run

100 bodyweight squats

BIBLIOGRAPHY

Arlinghaus, K. R., & Johnston, C. A. (2019). The Importance of Creating Habits and Routine. *American Journal of Lifestyle Medicine*, 142-144.

Army Public Health Center. (2016). *TECHNICAL INFORMATION PAPER NO. 12-054-0616: Foot Marching, Load Carriage, and Injury Risk*. Aberdeen Proving Grounds: TECHNICAL INFORMATION PAPER NO. 12-054-0616.

Askvik, E. O., Weel, F. v., & Meer, A. v. (2020). The Importance of Cursive Handwriting Over Typewriting for Learning in the Classroom: A High-Density EEG Study of 12-Year-Old Children and Young Adults. *Frontiers in Psychology*.

Beaven, C. M., Hopkins, W. G., Hansen, K. T., Wood, M. R., Cronin, J. B., & Lowe, T. E. (2018). Dose Effect of Caffeine on Testosterone and Cortisol Responses to Resistance Exercise. *International Journal of Sport Nutrition and Exercise Metabolism*, 131-141.

Bloch, A., Steckenrider, J., Zifchock, R., Freisinger, G., Bode, V., & Elkin-Frankston, S. (2023). *Effect of Fatigue on Movement Patterns During a Loaded Ruck March*. Military Medicine.

Carlson, M., & Jaenen, S. (2012). The development of a preselection physical fitness training program for Canadian Special Operations Regiment applicants. *Journal of Strength and Conditioning Research*.

CDC. (2021). *National Health and Nutrition Examination Survey*. Washington DC: CDC.

Cho, Y., Ryu, S.-H., Lee, B. R., Kim, K. H., Lee, E., & Choi, J. (2015). Effects of artificial light at night on human health: A literature review of observational and experimental studies applied to exposure assessment. *Chronobiology International*, 294-310.

Ebben, M. R., Yan, P., & Krieger, A. C. (2019). The effects of white noise on sleep and duration in individuals living in a high noise environment in New York City. *Sleep Medicine*, 256-259.

Farina, E. K., Thompson, L. A., Knapik, J. J., Pasiakos, S. M., McClung, J. M., & Lieberman, H. R. (2019). Physical performance, demographic, psychological, and physiological predictors of success in the U.S. Army Special Forces Assessment and Selection course. *Physiology & Behavior*.

Farina, E. K., Thompson, L. A., Knapik, J. J., Pasiakos, S. M., McClung, J. P., & Lieberman, H. R. (2022). Anthropometrics and Body Composition Predict Physical Performance and Selection to Attend Special Forces Training in United States Army Soldiers. *Military Medicine*.

Farrell, C., & Turgeon, D. R. (2023). Normal Versus Chronic Adaptations to Aerobic Exercise. *Nationa Library of Medicine*.

Gooley, J. J. (2017). Light Resetting and Entrainment of Human Circadian Rhythms.

In V. Kumar, *Biological Timekeeping: Clocks, Rhythms and Behaviour*. New Delhi: Springer.

Guth, L., & Roth, S. (2013). Genetic influence on athletic performance. *Current Opinions in Pediatrics*, 653-658.

Haghayegh, S., Khoshnevis, S., Smolensky, M., Diller, K., & Castriotta, R. (2019). Before-bedtime passive body heating by warm shower or bath to improve sleep: a systematic review and meta-analysis. *Sleep Medicine Review*, 124-135.

Halperin, D. (2014). Environmental noise and sleep disturbances: A threat to health? *Sleep Science*, 209-212.

Harding, E. C., Franks, N. P., & Wisden, W. (2020). Sleep and Thermoregulation. *Current Opinion in Physiology*, 7-13.

Harvard School of Public Health. (2023, November 30). *Processed Foods and Health*. Retrieved from Harvard School of Public Health : https://www.hsph.harvard.edu/nutritionsource/processed-foods/

Hellsten, Y., & Nyberg, M. (2015). Cardiovascular Adaptations to Exercise Training. *Comprehensive Physiology*, 1-32.

Hewitt, T. E. (2017). Prediction of Future Injury in Sport: Primary and Secondary Anterior Cruciate Ligament Injury Risk and Return to Sport as a Model. *Journal of Orthopaedic & Sports Physical Therapy*, 228-231.

Huberman, A. (2023). *NonSleep Deep Rest Protocol*. (A. Huberman, Performer)

Institute, A. (2023). *State of Play 2022*. Washington DC: Aspen Institute.

Jaramillo, A., Jaramillo, L., Castells, J., Beltran, A., Mora, N., Torres, S., . . . Santos, Y. (2023). Effectiveness of Creatine in Metabolic Performance: A Systematic Review and Meta-Analysis. *Cureus*.

Knapik, J. J., Harman, E. A., Steelman, R. A., & Graham, B. S. (2012). A Systematic Review of the Effects of Physical Training on Load Carriage Performance. *Journal of Strength and Conditioning Research*, 585-597.

Knapik, J., Reynolds, K., & Harman, E. (2004). *Soldier load carriage: historical, physiological, biomechanical, and medical aspects*. Mil Med.

Kraemer, W., Vescovi, J., Volek, J., Nindl, B., Newton, R., Patton, J., . . . Häkkinen, K. (2004). *Effects of concurrent resistance and aerobic training on load-bearing performance and the Army physical fitness test*. Military Medicine.

Krauchi, K., Werth, C. C., & Wirz-Justice, A. (1999). . Warm feet promote the rapid onset of sleep. Nature. 1999;401:36–37. *Nature*, 36-37.

Laury, D., & Tehrany, A. (2019). VO 2 Max Improvement of 96% in a Non-Elite Recreational Athlete over 24 Months. *The Surgery Journal*, 25-27.

Longo, U. G., Candela, V., Berton, A., Salvatore, G., Guarnieri, A., DeAngelis, J., . . . Denaro, V. (2019). Genetic basis of rotator cuff injury: a systematic review. *BMG MEdical Genetics*.

Lovallo, W. R., Whitsett, T. L., al'Absi, M., Sung, B. H., Vincent, A. S., & Wilson, M. F. (2005). Caffeine stimulation of cortisol secretion across the waking hours in relation to caffeine intake levels. *Psychosomatic Medicine*, 734-739.

MacInnis, M. J., & Gibala, M. J. (2017). Physiological adaptations to interval training and the role of exercise intensity. *The Journal of Physiology*, 2915-2930.

Maladouangdock, J. (2014). *The Role of Strength and Power in High Intensity Military Relevant Tasks*. University of Connecticut .

Medic, G., Wille, M., & Hemels, M. E. (2017). Short- and long-term health consequences of sleep disruption. *National Library of Medicine*, 151-161.

Milner, C., & Cote, K. (2009). Benefits of napping in healthy adults: impact of nap length, time of day, age, and experience with napping. *Journal of Sleep Research*.

NATO's Research & Technology Organization. (2009). *Optimizing Operational Physical Fitness*. Neuilly: NATO.

Okamoto-Mizuno, K., & Mizuno, K. (2012). Effects of thermal environment on sleep and circadian rhythm. *Journal of Physiological Anthropology*.

Orr, R., & Pope, R. (2015). Optimizing the Physical Training of Military Trainees. *Strength and Conditioning Journal*, 53-59.

Orr, R., Pope, R., Johnston, V., & Coyle, J. (2010). Load carriage: minimising soldierinjuries through physical conditioning –a narrative review. *Journal of Military and Veterans' Health*, 31-38.

Poel, D. (2016). *THE EFFECTS OF MILITARY STYLE RUCK MARCHING ON LOWER EXTREMITY LOADING*. The University of Wisconsin-Milwaukee.

Reddy, S., Reddy, V., & Sharma, S. (2023). Physiology, Circadian Rhythm. *Nationla Library of Medicine*.

Rosekind, M. R., Smith, R. M., Miller, D. l., Co, E. l., Gregory, K. B., Webbon, L. l., . . . Lebacqz, J. V. (1995). Alertness management: strategic naps in operational settings. *Journal of Sleep Medicine*.

Ross, J. (1993). Medial tibial stress syndrome in military recruits. *Ausstralian Military Medicine*, 17-18.

Schalkwijk, F. J., Sauter, C., Hoedlmoser, K., Heib, D. P., Klösch, G., Moser, D., . . . Schabus, M. (2017). The effect of daytime napping and full-night sleep on the consolidation of declarative and procedural information. *Journal of Sleep Research*.

Scialoia, D., & Swartzendruber, A. (2020). The R.I.C.E Protocol is a MYTH: A Review andRecommendations. *The Sport Journal*, 1-19.

Silvani, M. I., Werder, R., & Perret, C. (2022). The influence of blue light on sleep, performance and wellbeing in young adults: A systematic review. *Frontiers in Physiology* .

Singer, L., & Alexander, P. (2016). Reading Across Mediums: Effects of Reading Digital and Print Texts on Comprehension and Calibration. *The Journal of Experimental Education*, 155-172.

Sletten, T. L., Weaver, M. D., Foster, R. G., Gozal, D., Klerman, E. B., Rajaratnam, S. M., . . . Ture, F. W. (2023). The importance of sleep regularity: a consensus statement of the National Sleep Foundation sleep timing and variability panel. *Sleep Health*, 801-820.

Thakkar, M. M., Sharma, R., & Sahota, P. (2015). Alcohol disrupts sleep homeostasis. *Sleep*.

Umejima, K., Ibaraki, T., Yamazaki, T., & Sakai, K. L. (2021). Paper Notebooks vs. Mobile Devices: Brain Activation Differences During Memory Retrieval. *Frontiers in Behavioral Neuroscience*.

Uniformed Services University. (2023). *Load carriage strategies to improve military fitness*. Retrieved from Human Performance Resources by CHAMP: https://www. hprc-online.org/physical-fitness/training-performance/load-carriage-strategies-improve-military-fitness

Velky, J. (1990). Special Forces Assessment and Selection. *Special Warfare*, 12-15.

Wu, S.-H., Chen, K.-L., Hsu, C., Chen, H.-C., Chen, J.-Y., Yu, S.-Y., & Shiu, Y.-J. (2022). Creatine Supplementation for Muscle Growth: A Scoping Review of Randomized Clinical Trials from 2012 to 2021. *Nutrients*, .

Zuraikat, F. M., Wood, R. A., Barragán, R., & St-Onge, M.-P. (2021). Sleep and Diet: Mounting Evidence of a Cyclical Relationship. *Annual Reveiw of Nutrition*

PERFECT WEEK - DAY 1
Date: 12 AUG
Focus: Strength

SLEEP   Total Time   7.5

Quality   1   2   3   4 (5)

MOBILITY Mobility 1

STRENGTH   85% 1RM   4 Sets   8-10 Reps

Squat 215 / 10   215 / 10   215 / 10   215 / 8

Deadlift 295 / 10   295 / 10   295 / 10   295 / 10

OHP 115 / 10   115 / 10   115 / 10   115 / 10

2-4 minutes rest between sets

EMERGING LIMITATIONS: Left shoulder is tight

EMERGING CAPABILITIES: Hips are good now, keep working

NUTRITION   GOAL

TOTAL CALORIES: 2100   2300

GRAMS OF PROTEIN: 150   200

HYDRATION: 100 oz   100

READING: Supple Like a Leopard, shoulder chapter

RESEARCH: Find a PT for shoulder

PERFECT WEEK - DAY 2

Date: 13 AUG *Stayed up watching football. Stupid mistake*

Focus: Endurance

SLEEP Total Time _____ 5 _____

Quality   1   2   (3)   4   5

MOBILITY Mobility 2

ENDURANCE

	30 Min - Z2	30 Min - Z3
Mileage:	3.31	3.5
Avg HR:	130	150

Totally gassed. Couldn't catch breath

Conditions

Temperature:	70
Humidity:	65%
Time of Day:	0830

Socks: Asics   Shoes: Roclite

Hotspots: none

NUTRITION

		GOAL
TOTAL CALORIES:	2300	2300
GRAMS OF PROTEIN:	200	200
HYDRATION:	150	100

READING: Supple like a Leopard

RESEARCH: Shoulder mobility stuff

PERFECT WEEK - DAY 3

Date: 14 AUG
Focus: Strength

SLEEP   Total Time _____ 7.5 _____

Quality   1   2   3   4   (5)

Good sleep

MOBILITY   Mobility 1

STRENGTH   85% 1RM   4 Sets   8-10 Reps

Bench   19d.   10.   19b.   10.   19d.   10.   19d.   10

Row   16d.   10.   16b.   10.   16b.   10.   16b.   10

Shrug   115/.   10.   115/   10.   115/   10.   115/   10

2-4 minutes rest between sets

NUTRITION   GOAL

TOTAL CALORIES: 2100   2300

GRAMS OF PROTEIN: 150 need more protein   200

HYDRATION: 100 oz   100

READING: The Ugly American (why is this on the list?)

RESEARCH: Dept of State structure

PERFECT WEEK - DAY 4

Date: 15 AUG

Focus: Endurance

SLEEP   Total Time   8

              Quality   1   2   3   4   (5)

MOBILITY   Mobility 2

ENDURANCE

                              60 min run   Zone 2
                   Mileage: 6.8   Amazing run.
                   Avg HR: 132   Felt great

Conditions   Temperature: 71
                  Humidity: 70%
               Time of Day: 0600

Socks: Asics   Shoes: Brooks

Hotspots: none

NUTRITION   GOAL
         TOTAL CALORIES: 2100   2300
        GRAMS OF PROTEIN: 200   200
              HYDRATION: 100 oz   100

READING: Ugly American - Great book!

RESEARCH: Dept of State culture - why?

Date:

SLEEP   Total Time   7.5

            Quality

MOBILITY

    obility 1

STRENGTH   4 Sets   8-10 Reps

Squat	15	10	215	10	215	10	215	10
Deadlift								
OHP	115	10	115	10	115	10	115	10

NUTRITION   2100   2300

READING: 5 Years to freedom

RESEARCH

PERFECT WEEK - DAY 6
Date: 17 Aug
Focus: Skills

SLEEP Total Time   8 hrs

Quality   1   2   3   4   (5)

Hot shower is perfect. Slept amazing!

MOBILITY   Mobility 1 as Rx

SKILLS   From Menu

Rope Climbing x 5

Mantling x 5

Handstands x 10

Box Jumps - 3 x 15 @ 24inches

Dynamic Landing – 3 x 15 @ 24inches

Pistol Squats – 3 x 10 each leg

Jump Rope – 3 x 1 min

Shuffle runs – lateral, 20 sets

NUTRITION

		GOAL
TOTAL CALORIES:	2100	2300
GRAMS OF PROTEIN:	150	200
HYDRATION:	100 oz	100

READING: 5 Years to Freedom – Holy shit, this is amazing!

RESEARCH: What happened to Nick Rowe?

PERFECT WEEK - DAY 7
Date: 18 Aug
Focus: Rest

SLEEP   Total Time   7.5

Quality   1   2   3   4   (5)

MOBILITY

SUMMARY	SLEEP	CALORIES	PROTEIN	HYDRATION
Day 1	7.5	2300	150	
Day 2	5	2300	200	
Day 3	7.5	2100	150	
Day 4	8	2100	200	
Day 5	7.5	2100	150	
Day 6	7.5	2100	150	
Day 7	7.5	2300	150	

EMERGING LIMITATIONS: Need more protein

EMERGING CAPABILITIES: Sleep = Performance

NUTRITION   GOAL

TOTAL CALORIES: 2300   2300

GRAMS OF PROTEIN: 150   200

HYDRATION: 100 oz   100

NEXT WEEK TRAINING FOCUS: More consistent sleep, work

on shoulder mobility. Consistsency!!

Functional Movement Screening

0: You feel any pain at all
1: You can do the move, but not very well
2. You can do the move, but you need to compensate in some way.
3. You can perfectly master the move.

DEEP SQUAT   0   1   2   3

- Hold a dowel rod above your head. Then, squat as low as possible while keeping good form (head looking forward, chest upright, knees pointing forward).
- The goal is for your upper torso to be parallel with your shins and knees and dowel aligned over your feet.

INLINE LUNGE   0   1   2   3

- Hold the dowel behind your back with one hand near your neck and the other toward your lower back. Then, with your feet about hip-width apart and facing forward, step one foot back and lower it until it hits the floor. Use a balance pad for extra support if you need it.

- You're looking for the dowel to stay in place. Your torso to remain still, and your feet to face forward as your back knee lowers.

HURDLE STEP   0   1   2   3

- Hold the dowel across your shoulders in front of a hurdle. Now, step over the hurdle with one leg, touching the heel to the floor. Return to starting position. Then, repeat on the other side.

- You're looking for balance and for your upper body to remain neutral as you move your legs.

SHOULDER MOBILITY   0   1   2   3

- Reach your hands behind your back simultaneously, putting one over your shoulder and the other around your back reaching up. Repeat on the other side.
- Your goal is to get your hands as close together as possible.

ACTIVE STRAIGHT LEG RAISE   0   1   2   3

- Lie on your back with your arms at your sides. Raise one leg as high as you can while keeping your knee straight. The other leg remains on the floor.
- You're looking at how high you can raise your leg while keeping your other leg on the floor.

TRUNK STABILITY PUSH UP   0   1   2   3

- Get in a plank position and perform a push-up, going as far to the ground as possible before pushing yourself back into starting position. Cushion your hands using a yoga foam wedge block.

- Your goal is to get your chest to the ground and back up while keeping your body in a straight line.

ROTATIONAL STABILITY   0   1   2   3

- Put your knees down, so you are on all fours. Simultaneously raise your right leg and arm until they are parallel to the floor. Next, touch your right elbow to your right knee. Extend your arm and leg again, then put them on the floor before repeating on the left side.

- Your goal is to keep your elbow aligned with your knee and to do the move without twisting your torso. Pay attention to the differences between your left and right sides.

WEEK 1 - SUMMARY

This week is all about establishing baselines metrics across all of the domains that we will train. In order to determine how much progress that we are making, we need data to establish where we started. Many of these events, or parts of these events, will be humbling and eye-opening. Good. You have to start somewhere and this is where we start. You may also do quite well on some events. That good and will allow you prioritize other domains while maintaining these areas. Faster than the strongest lifter, stronger than the fastest runner.

Be diligent in recording your sleep, nutrition, and ancillary goals. Part of this week is figuring out how this journal works and figuring out how you can maximize its potential. You'll start to develop your own shorthand for notes and you might even add a few metrics. This is important because developing strong self-awareness is critical for success at SFAS.

DAY 1	FMS	Functional Movement Screening
DAY 2	PFA	Physical Fitness Assessment
DAY 3	1RM	1 Repetition Maximum Lift
DAY 4	5 MILE RUN	5 Mile Run
DAY 5	RUCK	12 Mile Ruck Assessment
DAY 6	MOBILITY PREP	Mobility Routine Development
DAY 7	REST	Rest, Journal, Plan, Meal Prep

If you can prep your meals for the week, it will make cramming in all of your calories and protein much easier. Remember, if you don't fuel your prep appropriately you're simply wasting all of that physical effort. Gains are made in the kitchen and the bedroom.

Take some time each week to think about your training goals. Maybe your goal is to simply do all of the reps and all of the exercises. Good. Maybe your goal is to do that AND get 8 hours of sleep every night. Better. Maybe your goal is to do all of that AND all of your protein and no booze and...and...and. Even better. Start building these habits now.

WEEK 1 - DAY 1
Date:
Focus: Functional Movement Screening

SLEEP   Total Time _____

            Quality   1   2   3   4   5

DEEP SQUAT	0	1	2	3
INLINE LUNGE	0	1	2	3
HURDLE STEP	0	1	2	3
SHOULDER MOBILITY	0	1	2	3
ACTIVE STRAIGHT LEG RAISE	0	1	2	3
TRUNK STABILITY PUSH UP	0	1	2	3
ROTATIONAL STABILITY	0	1	2	3

0: You feel any pain at all

1: You can do the move, but not very well

2. You can do the move, but you need to compensate in some way.

3. You can perfectly master the move.

Height: [＿＿＿＿＿]
Weight: [＿＿＿＿＿]

NUTRITION   GOAL

        TOTAL CALORIES: _____ _____

      GRAMS OF PROTEIN: _____ _____

            HYDRATION: _____ _____

READING: _____

RESEARCH: _____

WEEK 1 - DAY 2
Date:
Focus: PHYSICAL FITNESS ASSESSMENT

SLEEP   Total Time _____
            Quality   1   2   3   4   5

PFA

HRPU	
PLANK	
PULL-UPS	
2 MILE RUN	

EMERGING LIMITATIONS: _____

EMERGING CAPABILITIES: _____

NUTRITION   GOAL
        TOTAL CALORIES: _____ ____
      GRAMS OF PROTEIN: _____ ____
             HYDRATION: _____ ____

READING: _____

RESEARCH: _____

WEEK 1 - DAY 3
Date:
Focus: ESTABLISH 1 REP MAX

SLEEP   Total Time   _____

           Quality   1   2   3   4   5

MOBILITY

STRENGTH

                SQUAT _____

           DEADLIFT _____

              BENCH _____

                 ROW _____

              SHRUG _____

                 OHP _____

NUTRITION   GOAL

    TOTAL CALORIES: _____ _____

  GRAMS OF PROTEIN: _____ _____

        HYDRATION: _____ _____

READING: _____

RESEARCH: _____

WEEK 1 – DAY 4
Date:
Focus: 5 MILE RUN

SLEEP   Total Time   _____

                Quality   1   2   3   4   5

MOBILITY

5 MILE RUN

                    TIME _____

         AVERAGE HR: _____

Your time is your time. In your mind you will be chasing 35 minutes. It might take you 70. So be it, this is a start point. Run your run, record your time.

Conditions
    Temperature: _____
       Humidity: _____
     Time of Day: _____

SHOES _____
SOCKS _____
HOT SPOTS _____
PAIN POINTS _____

NUTRITION   GOAL

       TOTAL CALORIES: _____ ____
    GRAMS OF PROTEIN: _____ ____
          HYDRATION: _____ ____

READING: _____

RESEARCH: _____

WEEK 1 – DAY 5
Date:
Focus: RUCK ASSESSMENT

SLEEP   Total Time   _____

Quality   1   2   3   4   5

RUCK   Up to 12 Miles   35 pounds   Go as far and as
fast as you can
without injuring
yourself.

TIME   _____

AVERAGE HR: _____

Conditions

Temperature: _____

Humidity: _____

Time of Day: _____

BOOTS   _____

SOCKS   _____

HOT SPOTS   _____

PAIN POINTS   _____

NUTRITION   GOAL

TOTAL CALORIES: _____   _____

GRAMS OF PROTEIN: _____   _____

HYDRATION: _____   _____

READING: _____

RESEARCH: _____

WEEK 1 - DAY 6
Date:
Focus: MOBILITY ROUTINE DEVELOPMENT

SLEEP   Total Time   _____

                 Quality   1   2   3   4   5

MOBILITY

NUTRITION   GOAL

             TOTAL CALORIES: _____ _____

      GRAMS OF PROTEIN: _____ _____

                 HYDRATION: _____ _____

WEEK 1 - DAY 7
Date:
Focus: Rest

SLEEP   Total Time   _____

Quality   1   2   3   4   5

MOBILITY

SUMMARY	SLEEP	CALORIES	PROTEIN	HYDRATION
Day 1				
Day 2				
Day 3				
Day 4				
Day 5				
Day 6				
Day 7				

EMERGING LIMITATIONS: _____

EMERGING CAPABILITIES: _____

NUTRITION   GOAL

TOTAL CALORIES: _____

GRAMS OF PROTEIN: _____

HYDRATION: _____

NEXT WEEK TRAINING FOCUS: _____

WEEK 2 - SUMMARY

The assessment week is over, now we start working. This is where we start to build and reinforce good habits. This is where we start to identify distractions and bad habits. You can screw something up once or twice, after that its deliberate. You either fix it or you don't want it fixed. Hold yourself accountable.

DAY 1	MOBILITY 1	STRENGTH WORK
DAY 2	MOBILITY 2	ENDURANCE WORK
DAY 3	MOBILITY 1	STRENGTH WORK
DAY 4	MOBILITY 2	ENDURANCE WORK
DAY 5	MOBILITY 1	STRENGTH WORK
DAY 6	MOBILITY 1 & 2	SKILLS & ENDURANCE
DAY 7		REST

Consistency is key. Practice does not make perfect, practice makes permanent. Don't practice suboptimal procedures.

120 minutes of total endurance work this week.

Everyone wants to be a Green Beret until it's time to do Green Beret shit. It's time.

WEEK 2 - DAY 1
Date:
Focus: Strength

SLEEP   Total Time   _____
             Quality   1   2   3   4   5

MOBILITY

STRENGTH   80% 1RM   3 Sets   10-15 Reps

SQUAT   Wt   /   Reps   Wt   /   Reps   Wt   /   Reps
_____   _____   _____

DEADLIFT   Wt   /   Reps   Wt   /   Reps   Wt   /   Reps
_____   _____   _____

OHP   Wt   /   Reps   Wt   /   Reps   Wt   /   Reps
_____   _____   _____

1-2 minutes rest between sets

EMERGING LIMITATIONS: _____

EMERGING CAPABILITIES: _____

NUTRITION   GOAL
            TOTAL CALORIES: _____   _____
          GRAMS OF PROTEIN: _____   _____
                 HYDRATION: _____   _____

READING: _____

RESEARCH: _____

WEEK 2 - DAY 2
Date:
Focus: Endurance

SLEEP   Total Time   _____
             Quality   1   2   3   4   5

MOBILITY

ENDURANCE   40 Minutes   Zone 2
                Mileage: _____
                Avg HR: _____

              Conditions
           Temperature: _____
             Humidity: _____
          Time of Day: _____

EMERGING LIMITATIONS: _____

EMERGING CAPABILITIES: _____

NUTRITION   GOAL
        TOTAL CALORIES: _____ _____
      GRAMS OF PROTEIN: _____ _____
            HYDRATION: _____ _____

READING: _____

RESEARCH: _____

WEEK 2 - DAY 3
Date:
Focus: Strength

SLEEP   Total Time   _____

              Quality   1   2   3   4   5

MOBILITY

STRENGTH   80% 1RM   3 Sets   10-15 Reps

Bench Wt / Reps Wt / Reps Wt / Reps

Row Wt / Reps Wt / Reps Wt / Reps

Shrug Wt / Reps Wt / Reps Wt / Reps

1-2 minutes rest between sets

EMERGING LIMITATIONS: _____

EMERGING CAPABILITIES: _____

NUTRITION   GOAL

        TOTAL CALORIES: _____ _____

     GRAMS OF PROTEIN: _____ _____

           HYDRATION: _____ _____

READING: _____

RESEARCH: _____

WEEK 2 - DAY 4
Date:
Focus: Endurance

SLEEP   Total Time   _____
                Quality   1   2   3   4   5

MOBILITY

ENDURANCE   10 Min - Z2   30 Min - Z3
              Mileage: _____ _____
              Avg HR: _____ _____

            Conditions
          Temperature: _____
            Humidity: _____
         Time of Day: _____

EMERGING LIMITATIONS: _____

EMERGING CAPABILITIES: _____

NUTRITION   GOAL
         TOTAL CALORIES: _____ _____
      GRAMS OF PROTEIN: _____ _____
             HYDRATION: _____ _____

READING: _____

RESEARCH: _____

WEEK 2 - DAY 5

Date:

Focus: Strength

SLEEP   Total Time   _____

Quality   1   2   3   4   5

MOBILITY

STRENGTH   80% 1RM   3 Sets   10-15 Reps

SQUAT   Wt   /   Reps   Wt   /   Reps   Wt   /   Reps
_____

DEADLIFT   Wt   /   Reps   Wt   /   Reps   Wt   /   Reps
_____

OHP   Wt   /   Reps   Wt   /   Reps   Wt   /   Reps
_____

1-2 minutes rest between sets

EMERGING LIMITATIONS: _____

EMERGING CAPABILITIES: _____

NUTRITION   GOAL

TOTAL CALORIES: _____   _____

GRAMS OF PROTEIN: _____   _____

HYDRATION: _____   _____

READING: _____

RESEARCH: _____

WEEK 2 - DAY 6
Date:
Focus: Skills & Endurance

SLEEP   Total Time   _____
                Quality   1   2   3   4   5

MOBILITY

SKILLS

Pick 8 skills from the menu. Your set must include rope climb. Do a total of 45 minutes of work.

ENDURANCE   40 Min - Z2
              Mileage: _____
              Avg HR: _____

EMERGING LIMITATIONS: _____

EMERGING CAPABILITIES: _____

NUTRITION   GOAL
        TOTAL CALORIES: _____ ____
     GRAMS OF PROTEIN: _____ ____
            HYDRATION: _____ ____

READING: _____

RESEARCH: _____

WEEK 2 – DAY 7
Date:
Focus: Rest

SLEEP   Total Time   _____

                Quality   1   2   3   4   5

MOBILITY

SUMMARY	SLEEP	CALORIES	PROTEIN	HYDRATION
Day 1				
Day 2				
Day 3				
Day 4				
Day 5				
Day 6				
Day 7				

EMERGING LIMITATIONS: _____

EMERGING CAPABILITIES: _____

NUTRITION   GOAL

           TOTAL CALORIES: _____ _____

        GRAMS OF PROTEIN: _____ _____

                  HYDRATION: _____ _____

NEXT WEEK TRAINING FOCUS: _____

_____

WEEK 3 - SUMMARY

We are getting into the groove now. You should be figuring out what time of day works best for each workout so that you are reducing obstacles to performance. Your sleep routine should be fully developed now.

DAY 1	MOBILITY 1	STRENGTH WORK
DAY 2	MOBILITY 2	ENDURANCE WORK
DAY 3	MOBILITY 1	STRENGTH WORK
DAY 4	MOBILITY 2	ENDURANCE WORK
DAY 5	MOBILITY 1	STRENGTH WORK
DAY 6	MOBILITY 2	ENDURANCE WORK
DAY 7		REST

This is what we do now. We aren't 'working out', we are training. We are training for SFAS. That is our purpose.

140 minutes of total endurance work.

Get up when you said you would, workout when you said you would, eat exactly what you said you would. Are you a man of your word or not?

WEEK 3 – DAY 1
Date:
Focus: Strength

SLEEP   Total Time   _____

          Quality   1   2   3   4   5

MOBILITY

STRENGTH   80% 1RM   3 Sets   10-15 Reps

Bench Wt / Reps Wt / Reps Wt / Reps
_____

Row Wt / Reps Wt / Reps Wt / Reps
_____

Shrug Wt / Reps Wt / Reps Wt / Reps
_____

1-2 minutes rest between sets

EMERGING LIMITATIONS: _____

EMERGING CAPABILITIES: _____

NUTRITION   GOAL
          TOTAL CALORIES: _____ _____
          GRAMS OF PROTEIN: _____ _____
          HYDRATION: _____ _____

READING: _____

RESEARCH: _____

WEEK 3 - DAY 2
Date:
Focus: Endurance

SLEEP   Total Time   _____
              Quality   1   2   3   4   5

MOBILITY

ENDURANCE   45 Minutes   Zone 2
              Mileage: _____
              Avg HR: _____

          Conditions
         Temperature: _____
           Humidity: _____
       Time of Day: _____

EMERGING LIMITATIONS: _____

EMERGING CAPABILITIES: _____

NUTRITION   GOAL
      TOTAL CALORIES: _____ _____
    GRAMS OF PROTEIN: _____ _____
         HYDRATION: _____ _____

READING: _____

RESEARCH: _____

WEEK 3 – DAY 3
Date:
Focus: Strength

SLEEP   Total Time _____

             Quality   1   2   3   4   5

MOBILITY

STRENGTH   80% 1RM   3 Sets   10-15 Reps

SQUAT Wt / Reps Wt / Reps Wt / Reps

DEADLIFT Wt / Reps Wt / Reps Wt / Reps

OHP Wt / Reps Wt / Reps Wt / Reps

1-2 minutes rest between sets

EMERGING LIMITATIONS: _____

EMERGING CAPABILITIES: _____

NUTRITION   GOAL

      TOTAL CALORIES: _____ _____

    GRAMS OF PROTEIN: _____ _____

          HYDRATION: _____ _____

READING: _____

RESEARCH: _____

WEEK 3 - DAY 4
Date:
Focus: Endurance

SLEEP   Total Time   _____
             Quality   1   2   3   4   5

MOBILITY

ENDURANCE   10 Min - Z2   35 Min - Z3
                Mileage: _____   _____
                Avg HR: _____   _____

                Conditions
             Temperature: _____
               Humidity: _____
             Time of Day: _____

EMERGING LIMITATIONS: _____

EMERGING CAPABILITIES: _____

NUTRITION   GOAL
        TOTAL CALORIES: _____   _____
      GRAMS OF PROTEIN: _____   _____
            HYDRATION: _____   _____

READING: _____

RESEARCH: _____

WEEK 3 - DAY 5
Date:
Focus: Strength

SLEEP   Total Time   _____

            Quality   1   2   3   4   5

MOBILITY

STRENGTH   80% 1RM   3 Sets   10-15 Reps

Bench   Wt   /   Reps   Wt   /   Reps   Wt   /   Reps

Row   Wt   /   Reps   Wt   /   Reps   Wt   /   Reps

Shrug   Wt   /   Reps   Wt   /   Reps   Wt   /   Reps

1-2 minutes rest between sets

EMERGING LIMITATIONS: _____

EMERGING CAPABILITIES: _____

NUTRITION   GOAL

             TOTAL CALORIES: _____ _____

       GRAMS OF PROTEIN: _____ _____

                  HYDRATION: _____ _____

READING: _____

RESEARCH: _____

WEEK 3 - DAY 6
Date:
Focus: Endurance

SLEEP   Total Time   _____
            Quality   1   2   3   4   5

MOBILITY

ENDURANCE   50 Minutes   Zone 2
                Mileage: _____
                Avg HR: _____

                Conditions
            Temperature: _____
              Humidity: _____
           Time of Day: _____

EMERGING LIMITATIONS: _____

EMERGING CAPABILITIES: _____

NUTRITION   GOAL
        TOTAL CALORIES: _____ _____
      GRAMS OF PROTEIN: _____ _____
            HYDRATION: _____ _____

READING: _____

RESEARCH: _____

WEEK 3 - DAY 7
Date:
Focus: Rest

SLEEP   Total Time   _____
           Quality   1   2   3   4   5

MOBILITY

SUMMARY	SLEEP	CALORIES	PROTEIN	HYDRATION
Day 1				
Day 2				
Day 3				
Day 4				
Day 5				
Day 6				
Day 7				

EMERGING LIMITATIONS: _____

EMERGING CAPABILITIES: _____

NUTRITION   GOAL
        TOTAL CALORIES: _____ _____
    GRAMS OF PROTEIN: _____ _____
           HYDRATION: _____ _____

NEXT WEEK TRAINING FOCUS: _____
_____
_____

WEEK 4 - SUMMARY

We are moving at full speed now. All of your limitations are now known and you are specifically addressing them. Deliberate and intentional.

DAY 1	MOBILITY 1	STRENGTH WORK
DAY 2	MOBILITY 2	ENDURANCE WORK
DAY 3	MOBILITY 1	STRENGTH WORK
DAY 4	MOBILITY 2	SPEED WORK
DAY 5	MOBILITY 1	STRENGTH WORK
DAY 6	MOBILITY 2	ENDURANCE WORK
DAY 7		REST

You will execute your first speed session. It might feel like you are dying. Do it anyway. The vast majority of your cardio is still Zone 2, but we need to get faster. Faster than the strongest lifter.

160 minutes of total endurance work.

If you want to be a Green Beret, then act like it.

WEEK 4 - DAY 1
Date:
Focus: Strength

SLEEP   Total Time   _____

           Quality   1   2   3   4   5

MOBILITY

STRENGTH   80% 1RM   3 Sets   10-15 Reps

SQUAT Wt / Reps Wt / Reps Wt / Reps

DEADLIFT Wt / Reps Wt / Reps Wt / Reps

OHP Wt / Reps Wt / Reps Wt / Reps

1-2 minutes rest between sets

EMERGING LIMITATIONS: _____

EMERGING CAPABILITIES: _____

NUTRITION   GOAL

    TOTAL CALORIES: _____ _____

    GRAMS OF PROTEIN: _____ _____

    HYDRATION: _____ _____

READING: _____

RESEARCH: _____

WEEK 4 - DAY 2
Date:
Focus: Endurance

SLEEP   Total Time   _____
              Quality   1   2   3   4   5

MOBILITY

ENDURANCE   20 Min - Z2   30 Min - Z3
              Mileage: _____   _____
              Avg HR: _____   _____

              Conditions
              Temperature: _____
              Humidity: _____
              Time of Day: _____

EMERGING LIMITATIONS: _____

EMERGING CAPABILITIES: _____

NUTRITION   GOAL
              TOTAL CALORIES: _____ _____
              GRAMS OF PROTEIN: _____ _____
              HYDRATION: _____ _____

READING: _____

RESEARCH: _____

WEEK 4 - DAY 3

Date:

Focus: Strength

SLEEP   Total Time   _____

Quality   1   2   3   4   5

MOBILITY

STRENGTH   80% 1RM   3 Sets   10-15 Reps

Bench Wt / Reps Wt / Reps Wt / Reps

Row Wt / Reps Wt / Reps Wt / Reps

Shrug Wt / Reps Wt / Reps Wt / Reps

1-2 minutes rest between sets

EMERGING LIMITATIONS: _____

EMERGING CAPABILITIES: _____

NUTRITION   GOAL

TOTAL CALORIES: _____ _____

GRAMS OF PROTEIN: _____ _____

HYDRATION: _____ _____

READING: _____

RESEARCH: _____

WEEK 4 – DAY 4
Date:
Focus: Speed

SLEEP   Total Time   _____
             Quality   1   2   3   4   5

MOBILITY

ENDURANCE   10 Min – Z2   8 x 400 – Z4   1:1 means that if it
              Mileage: _____   1:1 work:rest   took you 2 minutes
              Avg HR: _____   to run the lap, then
                                                                you rest for 2
                                                                minutes

              Conditions   400 is one lap around
              Temperature: _____   a standard track.
              Humidity: _____
              Time of Day: _____

EMERGING LIMITATIONS: _____

EMERGING CAPABILITIES: _____

NUTRITION   GOAL
              TOTAL CALORIES: _____   _____
              GRAMS OF PROTEIN: _____   _____
              HYDRATION: _____   _____

READING: _____

RESEARCH: _____

WEEK 4 - DAY 5
Date:
Focus: Strength

SLEEP   Total Time   _____

                 Quality   1   2   3   4   5

MOBILITY

STRENGTH   80% 1RM   3 Sets   10-15 Reps

SQUAT   Wt / Reps   Wt / Reps   Wt / Reps

DEADLIFT   Wt / Reps   Wt / Reps   Wt / Reps

OHP   Wt / Reps   Wt / Reps   Wt / Reps

1-2 minutes rest between sets

EMERGING LIMITATIONS:

EMERGING CAPABILITIES:

NUTRITION   GOAL
          TOTAL CALORIES:
          GRAMS OF PROTEIN:
          HYDRATION:

READING:

RESEARCH:

WEEK 4 - DAY 6
Date:
Focus: Endurance

SLEEP   Total Time   _____
             Quality   1   2   3   4   5

MOBILITY

ENDURANCE   60 Minutes   Zone 2
            Mileage: _____
            Avg HR: _____

            Conditions
        Temperature: _____
          Humidity: _____
        Time of Day: _____

EMERGING LIMITATIONS: _____

EMERGING CAPABILITIES: _____

NUTRITION   GOAL
       TOTAL CALORIES: _____ _____
    GRAMS OF PROTEIN: _____ _____
          HYDRATION: _____ _____

READING: _____

RESEARCH: _____

WEEK 4 – DAY 7
Date:
Focus: Rest

SLEEP   Total Time   _____

               Quality   1   2   3   4   5

MOBILITY

SUMMARY	SLEEP	CALORIES	PROTEIN	HYDRATION
Day 1				
Day 2				
Day 3				
Day 4				
Day 5				
Day 6				
Day 7				

EMERGING LIMITATIONS: _____

EMERGING CAPABILITIES: _____

NUTRITION   GOAL

            TOTAL CALORIES: _____ _____

        GRAMS OF PROTEIN: _____ _____

                  HYDRATION: _____ _____

NEXT WEEK TRAINING FOCUS: _____

WEEK 5 - SUMMARY

We will do a quick assessment on Day 1 to measure any improvement on your PFT. If you are improving, then maintain your warm-up routine. If you are not improving then adjust your warm-up accordingly.

DAY 1	MOBILITY 1	ASSESSMENT
DAY 2	MOBILITY 2	ENDURANCE WORK
DAY 3	MOBILITY 1	STRENGTH WORK
DAY 4	MOBILITY 2	SPEED WORK
DAY 5	MOBILITY 1	STRENGTH WORK
DAY 6	MOBILITY 2	ENDURANCE WORK
DAY 7		REST

The FMS should reveal some improvements. If your mobility weaknesses are not improving, then you must adjust your mobility sessions accordingly.

180 minutes of total endurance work.

Results don't care about your feelings.

WEEK 5 - DAY 1
Date:
Focus: Assessment

PFA

HRPU	
PLANK	
PULL-UPS	
2 MILE RUN	

FMS

DEEP SQUAT	0	1	2	3
INLINE LUNGE	0	1	2	3
HURDLE STEP	0	1	2	3
SHOULDER MOBILITY	0	1	2	3
ACTIVE STRAIGHT LEG RAISE	0	1	2	3
TRUNK STABILITY PUSH UP	0	1	2	3
ROTATIONAL STABILITY	0	1	2	3

0: You feel any pain at all

1: You can do the move, but not very well

2. You can do the move, but you need to compensate in some way.

3. You can perfectly master the move.

NUTRITION   GOAL

TOTAL CALORIES: _____ _____

GRAMS OF PROTEIN: _____ _____

HYDRATION: _____ _____

READING: _____

RESEARCH: _____

WEEK 5 - DAY 2
Date:
Focus: Endurance

SLEEP   Total Time   _____
               Quality   1   2   3   4   5

MOBILITY

ENDURANCE   30 Min - Z2   30 Min - Z3
                   Mileage: _____ _____
                   Avg HR: _____ _____

         Conditions
         Temperature: _____
           Humidity: _____
        Time of Day: _____

EMERGING LIMITATIONS: _____

EMERGING CAPABILITIES: _____

NUTRITION   GOAL
        TOTAL CALORIES: _____ _____
     GRAMS OF PROTEIN: _____ _____
           HYDRATION: _____ _____

READING: _____

RESEARCH: _____

WEEK 5 - DAY 3
Date:
Focus: Strength

SLEEP   Total Time   _____

             Quality   1   2   3   4   5

MOBILITY

STRENGTH   80% 1RM   3 Sets   10-15 Reps

	Wt	/	Reps	Wt	/	Reps	Wt	/	Reps
Bench									
Row									
Shrug									

1-2 minutes rest between sets

EMERGING LIMITATIONS: _____

EMERGING CAPABILITIES: _____

NUTRITION   GOAL

           TOTAL CALORIES: _____

      GRAMS OF PROTEIN: _____

              HYDRATION: _____

READING: _____

RESEARCH: _____

WEEK 5 - DAY 4
Date:
Focus: Speed

SLEEP   Total Time   _____
              Quality   1   2   3   4   5

MOBILITY

ENDURANCE   20 Min - Z2   10 x 400 - Z4
              Mileage: _____   1:1 work:rest
              Avg HR: _____

              Conditions
              Temperature: _____
              Humidity: _____
              Time of Day: _____

EMERGING LIMITATIONS: _____

EMERGING CAPABILITIES: _____

NUTRITION   GOAL
              TOTAL CALORIES: _____ _____
              GRAMS OF PROTEIN: _____ _____
              HYDRATION: _____ _____

READING: _____

RESEARCH: _____

WEEK 5 – DAY 5
Date:
Focus: Strength

SLEEP   Total Time   _____

Quality   1   2   3   4   5

MOBILITY

STRENGTH   80% 1RM   3 Sets   10-15 Reps

SQUAT   Wt   /   Reps   Wt   /   Reps   Wt   /   Reps

DEADLIFT   Wt   /   Reps   Wt   /   Reps   Wt   /   Reps

OHP   Wt   /   Reps   Wt   /   Reps   Wt   /   Reps

1-2 minutes rest between sets

EMERGING LIMITATIONS: _____

EMERGING CAPABILITIES: _____

NUTRITION   GOAL

TOTAL CALORIES: _____

GRAMS OF PROTEIN: _____

HYDRATION: _____

READING: _____

RESEARCH: _____

WEEK 5 - DAY 6
Date:
Focus: Endurance

SLEEP   Total Time   _____
Quality   1   2   3   4   5

MOBILITY

ENDURANCE   60 Minutes   Zone 2
Mileage: _____
Avg HR: _____

Conditions
Temperature: _____
Humidity: _____
Time of Day: _____

EMERGING LIMITATIONS: _____

EMERGING CAPABILITIES: _____

NUTRITION   GOAL
TOTAL CALORIES: _____ ___
GRAMS OF PROTEIN: _____ ___
HYDRATION: _____ ___

READING: _____

RESEARCH: _____

WEEK 5 - DAY 7
Date:
Focus: Rest

SLEEP   Total Time   _____
            Quality   1   2   3   4   5

MOBILITY

SUMMARY	SLEEP	CALORIES	PROTEIN	HYDRATION
Day 1				
Day 2				
Day 3				
Day 4				
Day 5				
Day 6				
Day 7				

EMERGING LIMITATIONS: _____

EMERGING CAPABILITIES: _____

NUTRITION   GOAL
        TOTAL CALORIES: _____   ____
      GRAMS OF PROTEIN: _____   ____
            HYDRATION: _____   ____

NEXT WEEK TRAINING FOCUS: _____

_____
_____

MOBILITY WORKSHEET

MOBILITY WORKSHEET

WEEK 6 - SUMMARY

Deload endurance this week, but we transition to the heavier lifting schedule at 85% 1RM. You are not reestablishing your 1RM, you are simply increasing the percentage lift from your already established 1RM.

DAY 1	MOBILITY 1	STRENGTH WORK
DAY 2	MOBILITY 2	ENDURANCE WORK
DAY 3	MOBILITY 1	STRENGTH WORK
DAY 4	MOBILITY 1&2	SKILLS
DAY 5	MOBILITY 1	STRENGTH WORK
DAY 6	MOBILITY 2	ENDURANCE WORK
DAY 7		REST

We will introduce specific skills sessions now. You have a menu of 30 options. Pick the designated number of skills and practice them. Become useful. Become formidable. Take notes. Adjust your menu based on your performance.

150 minutes of total endurance work.

Build the foundation first, then worry about the walls.

WEEK 6 - DAY 1
Date:
Focus: Strength

SLEEP   Total Time   _____

              Quality   1   2   3   4   5

MOBILITY

STRENGTH   85% 1RM   4 Sets   8-10 Reps

Bench	Wt / Reps	Wt / Reps	Wt / Reps	Wt / Reps
Row	Wt / Reps	Wt / Reps	Wt / Reps	Wt / Reps
Shrug	Wt / Reps	Wt / Reps	Wt / Reps	Wt / Reps

2-4 minutes rest between sets

EMERGING LIMITATIONS: _____

EMERGING CAPABILITIES: _____

NUTRITION   GOAL

        TOTAL CALORIES: _____ _____

    GRAMS OF PROTEIN: _____ _____

           HYDRATION: _____ _____

READING: _____

RESEARCH: _____

WEEK 6 - DAY 2
Date:
Focus: Endurance

SLEEP   Total Time _____

            Quality   1   2   3   4   5

MOBILITY

ENDURANCE   40 Min - Z2   35 Min - Z3

             Mileage: _____ _____

             Avg HR: _____ _____

        Conditions

       Temperature: _____

         Humidity: _____

      Time of Day: _____

EMERGING LIMITATIONS: _____

EMERGING CAPABILITIES: _____

NUTRITION   GOAL

       TOTAL CALORIES: _____ _____

   GRAMS OF PROTEIN: _____ _____

          HYDRATION: _____ _____

READING: _____

RESEARCH: _____

WEEK 6 - DAY 3
Date:
Focus: Strength

SLEEP   Total Time   _____
            Quality   1   2   3   4   5

MOBILITY

STRENGTH   85% 1RM   4 Sets   8-10 Reps

Squat Wt / Reps Wt / Reps Wt / Reps Wt / Reps

Deadlift Wt / Reps Wt / Reps Wt / Reps Wt / Reps

OHP Wt / Reps Wt / Reps Wt / Reps Wt / Reps

2-4 minutes rest between sets

EMERGING LIMITATIONS: _____

EMERGING CAPABILITIES: _____

NUTRITION   GOAL
            TOTAL CALORIES: _____ _____
            GRAMS OF PROTEIN: _____ _____
            HYDRATION: _____ _____

READING: _____

RESEARCH: _____

WEEK 6 - DAY 4
Date:
Focus: Skills

SLEEP   Total Time   _____
              Quality   1   2   3   4   5

MOBILITY

 SKILLS   From Menu

Write down one story-worthy moment each day. In a month you'll have 30 stories.

EMERGING LIMITATIONS: _____

EMERGING CAPABILITIES: _____

NUTRITION   GOAL
              TOTAL CALORIES: _____ _____
              GRAMS OF PROTEIN: _____ _____
              HYDRATION: _____ _____

READING: _____

RESEARCH: _____

WEEK 6 - DAY 5
Date:
Focus: Strength

SLEEP   Total Time   _____

           Quality   1   2   3   4   5

MOBILITY

STRENGTH   85% 1RM   4 Sets   8-10 Reps

	Wt	/	Reps	Wt	/	Reps	Wt	/	Reps	Wt	/	Reps
Bench												
Row												
Shrug												

2-4 minutes rest between sets

EMERGING LIMITATIONS: _____

EMERGING CAPABILITIES: _____

NUTRITION   GOAL

            TOTAL CALORIES: _____

      GRAMS OF PROTEIN: _____

               HYDRATION: _____

READING: _____

RESEARCH: _____

WEEK 6 - DAY 6
Date:
Focus: Endurance

SLEEP   Total Time   _____
              Quality   1   2   3   4   5

MOBILITY

ENDURANCE   75 Minutes   Zone 2
                Mileage: _____
                Avg HR: _____

                Conditions
             Temperature: _____
                Humidity: _____
             Time of Day: _____

EMERGING LIMITATIONS: _____

EMERGING CAPABILITIES: _____

NUTRITION   GOAL
          TOTAL CALORIES: _____ _____
        GRAMS OF PROTEIN: _____ _____
              HYDRATION: _____ _____

READING: _____

RESEARCH: _____

WEEK 6 – DAY 7
Date:
Focus: Rest

SLEEP   Total Time   _____

            Quality   1   2   3   4   5

MOBILITY

SUMMARY	SLEEP	CALORIES	PROTEIN	HYDRATION
Day 1				
Day 2				
Day 3				
Day 4				
Day 5				
Day 6				
Day 7				

EMERGING LIMITATIONS: _____

EMERGING CAPABILITIES: _____

NUTRITION   GOAL

          TOTAL CALORIES: _____ _____

       GRAMS OF PROTEIN: _____ _____

              HYDRATION: _____ _____

NEXT WEEK TRAINING FOCUS: _____

_____

_____

WEEK 7 - SUMMARY

Deload week is over; we are going to put the boots to you this week. This will include more speed work. Your body is making the physiological adaptations in earnest now, so you should be feeling stronger and faster. Not much, but progress. Imagine where you will be in a few months?

DAY 1	MOBILITY 1	STRENGTH WORK
DAY 2	MOBILITY 2	ENDURANCE WORK
DAY 3	MOBILITY 1	STRENGTH WORK
DAY 4	MOBILITY 2	SPEED WORK
DAY 5	MOBILITY 1	STRENGTH WORK
DAY 6	MOBILITY 2	ENDURANCE WORK
DAY 7		REST

240 minutes of total endurance work.

No parent wishes for a weak son. No woman wishes for a weak man. No child wishes for a weak father. Live up to your duty and get stronger.

WEEK 7 - DAY 1
Date:
Focus: Strength

SLEEP   Total Time   _____
        Quality   1   2   3   4   5

MOBILITY

STRENGTH   85% 1RM   4 Sets   8-10 Reps

	Wt	/	Reps	Wt	/	Reps	Wt	/	Reps	Wt	/	Reps
Squat												
Deadlift												
OHP												

2-4 minutes rest between sets

EMERGING LIMITATIONS: _____

EMERGING CAPABILITIES: _____

NUTRITION   GOAL
    TOTAL CALORIES: _____ _____
    GRAMS OF PROTEIN: _____ _____
    HYDRATION: _____ _____

READING: _____

RESEARCH: _____

WEEK 7 - DAY 2
Date:
Focus: Endurance

<u>**SLEEP**</u>   Total Time   _____
                Quality   1   2   3   4   5

<u>**MOBILITY**</u>

<u>**ENDURANCE**</u>   40 Min - Z2   40 Min - Z3
             Mileage: _____ _____
             Avg HR: _____ _____

           <u>Conditions</u>
         Temperature: _____
            Humidity: _____
         Time of Day: _____

EMERGING LIMITATIONS: _____

EMERGING CAPABILITIES: _____

<u>**NUTRITION**</u>   GOAL
        TOTAL CALORIES: _____ _____
    GRAMS OF PROTEIN: _____ _____
           HYDRATION: _____ _____

READING: _____

RESEARCH: _____

WEEK 7 - DAY 3
Date:
Focus: Strength

SLEEP   Total Time   _____

                    Quality   1   2   3   4   5

MOBILITY

STRENGTH   85% 1RM   4 Sets   8-10 Reps

Bench Wt / Reps Wt / Reps Wt / Reps Wt / Reps

Row Wt / Reps Wt / Reps Wt / Reps Wt / Reps

Shrug Wt / Reps Wt / Reps Wt / Reps Wt / Reps

2-4 minutes rest between sets

EMERGING LIMITATIONS:

EMERGING CAPABILITIES:

NUTRITION   GOAL

        TOTAL CALORIES:

      GRAMS OF PROTEIN:

              HYDRATION:

READING:

RESEARCH:

SLEEP   Total Time _____

               Quality   1   2   3   4   5

MOBILITY

ENDURANCE   30 Min - Z2   6 x 800 - Z4   800 is two laps

               Mileage: _____   1:1 work:rest   around a standard

               Avg HR: _____   track.

               Conditions

               Temperature: _____

               Humidity: _____

               Time of Day: _____

EMERGING LIMITATIONS: _____

EMERGING CAPABILITIES: _____

NUTRITION   GOAL

        TOTAL CALORIES: _____ _____

      GRAMS OF PROTEIN: _____ _____

           HYDRATION: _____ _____

READING: _____

RESEARCH: _____

WEEK 7 - DAY 5
Date:
Focus: Strength

SLEEP   Total Time   _____

                  Quality   1   2   3   4   5

MOBILITY

STRENGTH   85% 1RM   4 Sets   8-10 Reps

Squat Wt / Reps Wt / Reps Wt / Reps Wt / Reps

Deadlift Wt / Reps Wt / Reps Wt / Reps Wt / Reps

OHP Wt / Reps Wt / Reps Wt / Reps Wt / Reps

2-4 minutes rest between sets

EMERGING LIMITATIONS: _____

EMERGING CAPABILITIES: _____

NUTRITION   GOAL

        TOTAL CALORIES: _____

      GRAMS OF PROTEIN: _____

           HYDRATION: _____

READING: _____

RESEARCH: _____

WEEK 7 - DAY 6
Date:
Focus: Endurance

SLEEP Total Time _____
Quality   1   2   3   4   5

MOBILITY

ENDURANCE   80 Minutes   Zone 2
Mileage: _____
Avg HR: _____

Conditions
Temperature: _____
Humidity: _____
Time of Day: _____

EMERGING LIMITATIONS: _____

EMERGING CAPABILITIES: _____

NUTRITION   GOAL
TOTAL CALORIES: _____ _____
GRAMS OF PROTEIN: _____ _____
HYDRATION: _____ _____

READING: _____

RESEARCH: _____

WEEK 7 - DAY 7
Date:
Focus: Rest

SLEEP   Total Time   _____

          Quality   1   2   3   4   5

MOBILITY

SUMMARY	SLEEP	CALORIES	PROTEIN	HYDRATION
Day 1				
Day 2				
Day 3				
Day 4				
Day 5				
Day 6				
Day 7				

EMERGING LIMITATIONS: _____

EMERGING CAPABILITIES: _____

NUTRITION   GOAL
          TOTAL CALORIES: _____ _____
       GRAMS OF PROTEIN: _____ _____
                HYDRATION: _____ _____

NEXT WEEK TRAINING FOCUS: _____

_____
_____

WEEK 8 – SUMMARY

No speed work, lots of Zone 2 and strength training. This is not a deload week, but it is a "standard" week of "regular training." No skills work, no speed work, just work. Get dialed back in to your core tasks. Faster, stronger.

DAY 1	MOBILITY 1	STRENGTH WORK
DAY 2	MOBILITY 2	ENDURANCE WORK
DAY 3	MOBILITY 1	STRENGTH WORK
DAY 4	MOBILITY 2	ENDURANCE WORK
DAY 5	MOBILITY 1	STRENGTH WORK
DAY 6	MOBILITY 2	ENDURANCE WORK
DAY 7		REST

270 minutes of total endurance work.

Good enough isn't good enough. Outwork the doubt.

WEEK 8 - DAY 1
Date:
Focus: Strength

SLEEP   Total Time   _____
            Quality   1   2   3   4   5

MOBILITY

STRENGTH   85% 1RM   4 Sets   8-10 Reps

Bench   Wt   /   Reps   Wt   /   Reps   Wt   /   Reps   Wt   /   Reps

Row   Wt   /   Reps   Wt   /   Reps   Wt   /   Reps   Wt   /   Reps

Shrug   Wt   /   Reps   Wt   /   Reps   Wt   /   Reps   Wt   /   Reps

2-4 minutes rest between sets

EMERGING LIMITATIONS: _____

EMERGING CAPABILITIES: _____

NUTRITION   GOAL
            TOTAL CALORIES: _____   _____
        GRAMS OF PROTEIN: _____   _____
                HYDRATION: _____   _____

READING: _____

RESEARCH: _____

WEEK 8 - DAY 2
Date:
Focus: Endurance

SLEEP   Total Time   _____

             Quality   1   2   3   4   5

MOBILITY

ENDURANCE   45 Min - Z2   45 Min - Z3

              Mileage: _____ _____

              Avg HR: _____ _____

            Conditions

          Temperature: _____

            Humidity: _____

        Time of Day: _____

EMERGING LIMITATIONS: _____

EMERGING CAPABILITIES: _____

NUTRITION   GOAL

      TOTAL CALORIES: _____ ____

    GRAMS OF PROTEIN: _____ ____

         HYDRATION: _____ ____

READING: _____

RESEARCH: _____

WEEK 8 - DAY 3
Date:
Focus: Strength

SLEEP   Total Time   _____
Quality   1   2   3   4   5

MOBILITY

STRENGTH   85% 1RM   4 Sets   8-10 Reps

Squat   Wt   /   Reps   Wt   /   Reps   Wt   /   Reps   Wt   /   Reps
_____

Deadlift   Wt   /   Reps   Wt   /   Reps   Wt   /   Reps   Wt   /   Reps
_____

OHP   Wt   /   Reps   Wt   /   Reps   Wt   /   Reps   Wt   /   Reps
_____

2-4 minutes rest between sets

EMERGING LIMITATIONS: _____

EMERGING CAPABILITIES: _____

NUTRITION   GOAL
TOTAL CALORIES: _____   _____
GRAMS OF PROTEIN: _____   _____
HYDRATION: _____   _____

READING: _____

RESEARCH: _____

WEEK 8 - DAY 4
Date:
Focus: Endurance

SLEEP   Total Time   _____
             Quality   1   2   3   4   5

MOBILITY

ENDURANCE   90 Minutes   Zone 2
                Mileage: _____
                Avg HR: _____

                Conditions
            Temperature: _____
               Humidity: _____
            Time of Day: _____

EMERGING LIMITATIONS: _____

EMERGING CAPABILITIES: _____

NUTRITION   GOAL
        TOTAL CALORIES: _____ _____
      GRAMS OF PROTEIN: _____ _____
             HYDRATION: _____ _____

READING: _____

RESEARCH: _____

WEEK 8 – DAY 5
Date:
Focus: Strength

SLEEP Total Time _____
Quality   1   2   3   4   5

MOBILITY

STRENGTH   85% 1RM   4 Sets   8-10 Reps

Bench   Wt / Reps Wt / Reps Wt / Reps Wt / Reps

Row   Wt / Reps Wt / Reps Wt / Reps Wt / Reps

Shrug   Wt / Reps Wt / Reps Wt / Reps Wt / Reps

2-4 minutes rest between sets

EMERGING LIMITATIONS: _____

EMERGING CAPABILITIES: _____

NUTRITION   GOAL
            TOTAL CALORIES: _____ _____
        GRAMS OF PROTEIN: _____ _____
                HYDRATION: _____ _____

READING: _____

RESEARCH: _____

WEEK 8 - DAY 6
Date:
Focus: Endurance

SLEEP   Total Time   _____
               Quality   1   2   3   4   5

MOBILITY

ENDURANCE   90 Minutes   Zone 2
               Mileage: _____
               Avg HR: _____

               Conditions
           Temperature: _____
             Humidity: _____
          Time of Day: _____

EMERGING LIMITATIONS: _____

EMERGING CAPABILITIES: _____

NUTRITION   GOAL
          TOTAL CALORIES: _____ _____
      GRAMS OF PROTEIN: _____ _____
             HYDRATION: _____ _____

READING: _____

RESEARCH: _____

WEEK 8 - DAY 7
Date:
Focus: Rest

SLEEP   Total Time   _____

             Quality   1   2   3   4   5

MOBILITY

SUMMARY	SLEEP	CALORIES	PROTEIN	HYDRATION
Day 1				
Day 2				
Day 3				
Day 4				
Day 5				
Day 6				
Day 7				

EMERGING LIMITATIONS: _____

EMERGING CAPABILITIES: _____

NUTRITION   GOAL

        TOTAL CALORIES: _____ _____

      GRAMS OF PROTEIN: _____ _____

             HYDRATION: _____ _____

NEXT WEEK TRAINING FOCUS: _____
_____
_____

WEEK 9 - SUMMARY

We are closing out Phase 1 this week. Next week you will assess each domain and if you have progressed enough you get to continue to Phase 2. You get to earn the privilege if rucking.

DAY 1	MOBILITY 1	STRENGTH WORK
DAY 2	MOBILITY 2	ENDURANCE WORK
DAY 3	MOBILITY 1	STRENGTH WORK
DAY 4	MOBILITY 2	ENDURANCE WORK
DAY 5	MOBILITY 1	STRENGTH WORK
DAY 6	MOBILITY 2	SKILLS WORK
DAY 7		REST

Make this week count.

Mathematically, this is also an endurance deload week.

How long are you going to wait before you demand the best
from yourself?   - Epictetus

WEEK 9 - DAY 1
Date:
Focus: Strength

SLEEP Total Time _____
Quality   1   2   3   4   5

MOBILITY

STRENGTH   85% 1RM   4 Sets   8-10 Reps

Squat Wt / Reps Wt / Reps Wt / Reps Wt / Reps

Deadlift Wt / Reps Wt / Reps Wt / Reps Wt / Reps

OHP Wt / Reps Wt / Reps Wt / Reps Wt / Reps

2-4 minutes rest between sets

EMERGING LIMITATIONS: _____

EMERGING CAPABILITIES: _____

NUTRITION   GOAL
TOTAL CALORIES: _____ _____
GRAMS OF PROTEIN: _____ _____
HYDRATION: _____ _____

READING: _____

RESEARCH: _____

WEEK 9 - DAY 2
Date:
Focus: Endurance

SLEEP   Total Time   _____
               Quality   1   2   3   4   5

MOBILITY

ENDURANCE

	30 Min - Z2	30 Min - Z3
Mileage:	_____	_____
Avg HR:	_____	_____

Conditions   Temperature: _____
                 Humidity: _____
            Time of Day: _____

NUTRITION   GOAL
        TOTAL CALORIES: _____ _____
      GRAMS OF PROTEIN: _____ _____
            HYDRATION: _____ _____

READING: _____

RESEARCH: _____

WEEK 9 - DAY 3
Date:
Focus: Strength

SLEEP   Total Time   _____
               Quality   1   2   3   4   5

MOBILITY

STRENGTH   85% 1RM   4 Sets   8-10 Reps

Bench   Wt   /   Reps   Wt   /   Reps   Wt   /   Reps   Wt   /   Reps

Row   Wt   /   Reps   Wt   /   Reps   Wt   /   Reps   Wt   /   Reps

Shrug   Wt   /   Reps   Wt   /   Reps   Wt   /   Reps   Wt   /   Reps

2-4 minutes rest between sets

NUTRITION   GOAL
        TOTAL CALORIES: _____   _____
     GRAMS OF PROTEIN: _____   _____
           HYDRATION: _____   _____

READING: _____

RESEARCH: _____

WEEK 9 – DAY 4
Date:
Focus: Endurance

<u>SLEEP</u>   Total Time _____
          Quality   1   2   3   4   5

<u>MOBILITY</u>

<u>ENDURANCE</u>

                    60 min run   Zone 2
          Mileage: _____
          Avg HR: _____

<u>Conditions</u>   Temperature: _____
            Humidity: _____
          Time of Day: _____

<u>NUTRITION</u>   GOAL
        TOTAL CALORIES: _____ _____
        GRAMS OF PROTEIN: _____ _____
              HYDRATION: _____ _____

READING: _____

RESEARCH: _____

WEEK 9 - DAY 5

Date:

Focus: Strength

SLEEP   Total Time

_____

Quality   1   2   3   4   5

MOBILITY

STRENGTH   85% 1RM   4 Sets   8-10 Reps

Squat Wt / Reps Wt / Reps Wt / Reps Wt / Reps

_____

Deadlift Wt / Reps Wt / Reps Wt / Reps Wt / Reps

_____

OHP Wt / Reps Wt / Reps Wt / Reps Wt / Reps

_____

2-4 minutes rest between sets

EMERGING LIMITATIONS: _____

EMERGING CAPABILITIES: _____

NUTRITION   GOAL

TOTAL CALORIES: _____ _____

GRAMS OF PROTEIN: _____ _____

HYDRATION: _____ _____

READING: _____

RESEARCH: _____

WEEK 9 - DAY 6
Date:
Focus: Skills

SLEEP   Total Time   _____
            Quality   1   2   3   4   5

MOBILITY

SKILLS   From Menu

NUTRITION   GOAL
            TOTAL CALORIES: _____ _____
            GRAMS OF PROTEIN: _____ _____
            HYDRATION: _____ _____

READING: _____

RESEARCH: _____

WEEK 9 – DAY 7
Date:
Focus: Rest

SLEEP   Total Time   _____

                Quality   1   2   3   4   5

MOBILITY

SUMMARY	SLEEP	CALORIES	PROTEIN	HYDRATION
Day 1				
Day 2				
Day 3				
Day 4				
Day 5				
Day 6				
Day 7				

EMERGING LIMITATIONS: _____

EMERGING CAPABILITIES: _____

NUTRITION   GOAL

        TOTAL CALORIES: _____ _____

    GRAMS OF PROTEIN: _____ _____

            HYDRATION: _____ _____

NEXT WEEK TRAINING FOCUS: _____

_____

_____

WEEK 10 - SUMMARY
PHASE 1 ASSESSMENT

This week we test out of Phase 1 and start Phase 2 and it is all about re-establishing baseline metrics across all of the domains that we have been training so that we can see how far we have come...and decide if we are ready to proceed with this next phase or re-engage for a few weeks to meet the prerequisites. If you are unable to 1RM Bench Press .85x your BW, 1.25x BW 1RM Squat, and 1.5x BW 1RM Deadlift then you are not ready to proceed. Repeat the last 4 weeks. This program is not time driven, it is performance driven. Do not rush to failure.

DAY 1	FMS	Functional Movement Screening
DAY 2	PFA	Physical Fitness Assessment
DAY 3	1RM	1 Repetition Maximum Lift
DAY 4	5 MILE RUN	5 Mile Run
DAY 5	RUCK	12 Mile Ruck Assessment
DAY 6	MOBILITY PREP	Mobility Routine Development
DAY 7	REST	Rest, Journal, Plan, Meal Prep

Review that last 9 weeks of training journals and look for blank spots. There should be very few blank spots. Do you have a blank spot under the reading and research lines? Why? You have a comprehensive reading list. Do you enjoy a limited vocabulary, because people who don't read have limited vocabularies. Do you like being a boring conversationalist? Is there literally nothing that you wanted to research? An idea? A product? A technique? Nothing? Don't you have any intellectual curiosity? These are things that will help you become formidable.

Take copious notes about what socks, boots, and insoles you are wearing. Do the boots support you as desired...arches, Achilles, footbed? Are you getting hotspots?

If you're going to be elite, you have to do elite things.

WEEK 10 - DAY 1
Date:
Focus: Functional Movement Screening

SLEEP   Total Time   _____

Quality   1   2   3   4   5

DEEP SQUAT	0	1	2	3
INLINE LUNGE	0	1	2	3
HURDLE STEP	0	1	2	3
SHOULDER MOBILITY	0	1	2	3
ACTIVE STRAIGHT LEG RAISE	0	1	2	3
TRUNK STABILITY PUSH UP	0	1	2	3
ROTATIONAL STABILITY	0	1	2	3

0: You feel any pain at all

1: You can do the move, but not very well

2. You can do the move, but you need to compensate in some way.

3. You can perfectly master the move.

Height: _____
Weight: _____

NUTRITION   GOAL

TOTAL CALORIES: _____ _____

GRAMS OF PROTEIN: _____ _____

HYDRATION: _____ _____

READING: _____

RESEARCH: _____

WEEK 10 - DAY 2
Date:
Focus: PHYSICAL FITNESS ASSESSMENT

SLEEP   Total Time _____

Quality   1   2   3   4   5

PFA

HRPU	
PLANK	
PULL-UPS	
2 MILE RUN	

EMERGING LIMITATIONS: _____

EMERGING CAPABILITIES: _____

NUTRITION   GOAL

TOTAL CALORIES: _____ _____

GRAMS OF PROTEIN: _____ _____

HYDRATION: _____ _____

READING: _____

RESEARCH: _____

WEEK 10 – DAY 3
Date:
Focus: ESTABLISH 1 REP MAX

SLEEP   Total Time   _____
             Quality   1   2   3   4   5

MOBILITY

STRENGTH

SQUAT   _____

DEADLIFT   _____

BENCH   _____

ROW   _____

SHRUG   _____

OHP   _____

NUTRITION   GOAL
          TOTAL CALORIES: _____   _____
          GRAMS OF PROTEIN: _____   _____
          HYDRATION: _____   _____

READING: _____

RESEARCH: _____

SLEEP Total Time _____

Quality   1   2   3   4   5

MOBILITY

5 MILE RUN

TIME _____

AVERAGE HR: _____

Your time is your time. In your mind you will be chasing 35 minutes. You should see significant improvement from your last 5 miles run. Run your run, record your time. The data does not lie.

Conditions

Temperature: _____

Humidity: _____

Time of Day: _____

SHOES _____

SOCKS _____

HOT SPOTS _____

PAIN POINTS _____

NUTRITION   GOAL

TOTAL CALORIES: 2300   2300

GRAMS OF PROTEIN: 2300   2300

HYDRATION: 2300   2300

READING: _____

RESEARCH: _____

WEEK 10 - DAY 5
Date:
Focus: RUCK ASSESSMENT

SLEEP   Total Time   _____
              Quality   1   2   3   4   5

RUCK   12 miles   35 pounds
                    TIME   _____
              AVERAGE HR: _____

              Conditions
                Temperature: _____
                   Humidity: _____
                Time of Day: _____

BOOTS   _____
SOCKS   _____
HOT SPOTS   _____
PAIN POINTS   _____

NUTRITION   GOAL
        TOTAL CALORIES: _____   _____
      GRAMS OF PROTEIN: _____   _____
            HYDRATION: _____   _____

READING: _____

RESEARCH: _____

SLEEP   Total Time   _____
             Quality   1   2   3   4   5

Spend some time today redeveloping your mobility, warm-up, and movement prep routines. With the introduction of rucking, you may note some additional requirements.

EMERGING LIMITATIONS: _____

EMERGING CAPABILITIES: _____

NUTRITION   GOAL
        TOTAL CALORIES: _____ _____
      GRAMS OF PROTEIN: _____ _____
            HYDRATION: _____ _____

WEEK 10 - DAY 7
Date:
Focus: Rest

SLEEP   Total Time _____

            Quality   1   2   3   4   5

MOBILITY

SUMMARY	SLEEP	CALORIES	PROTEIN	HYDRATION
Day 1				
Day 2				
Day 3				
Day 4				
Day 5				
Day 6				
Day 7				

EMERGING LIMITATIONS: _____

EMERGING CAPABILITIES: _____

NUTRITION   GOAL

        TOTAL CALORIES: _____ _____

      GRAMS OF PROTEIN: _____ _____

             HYDRATION: _____ _____

NEXT WEEK TRAINING FOCUS: _____

MOBILITY WORKSHEET

WEEK 11 - SUMMARY

Phase 2 begins. The strength foundation is established. We will continue to grow this. The cardio foundation is established and now we can begin rucking. We will also begin incorporating some cognitive load into our conditioning sessions. Just follow the prompts we have provided. At the end of the day during your reflection you can assess and write down your results.

DAY 1	MOBILITY 1	STRENGTH WORK
DAY 2	MOBILITY 2	ENDURANCE WORK
DAY 3	MOBILITY 1	STRENGTH WORK
DAY 4	MOBILITY 2	ENDURANCE WORK
DAY 5	MOBILITY 1	STRENGTH WORK
DAY 6	MOBILITY 2	ENDURANCE & SPEED
DAY 7		REST

We are going to start rucking this Phase. If you are unable to complete 90 unbroken minutes of Zone 2 running then you are not ready to proceed. Repeat the last 4 weeks. if you are ready, we will start rucking slow with low weight. We are working to build some specific adaptations. We want our muscles to handle this novel load, we want to focus on technique, and we want to start to harden our feet. This takes time. Allow the process to work. Keep accurate and descriptive notes.

You have 3 rucks with 6 miles this week.

You will note that we do not prescribe a HR Zone goal for rucks. Concentrate on being as fast as you can without sacrificing technique.

You're going fail, a lot. Until you don't.

WEEK 11 – DAY 1
Date:
Focus: Strength

<u>SLEEP</u> Total Time _____
Quality   1   2   3   4   5

<u>MOBILITY</u>

<u>STRENGTH</u>   80% 1RM   3 Sets   10-15 Reps

Bench   Wt   /   Reps   Wt   /   Reps   Wt   /   Reps

Row   Wt   /   Reps   Wt   /   Reps   Wt   /   Reps

Shrug   Wt   /   Reps   Wt   /   Reps   Wt   /   Reps

1-2 minutes rest between sets

EMERGING LIMITATIONS: _____

EMERGING CAPABILITIES: _____

<u>NUTRITION</u>   GOAL
TOTAL CALORIES: _____
GRAMS OF PROTEIN: _____
HYDRATION: _____

READING: _____

RESEARCH: _____

WEEK 11 - DAY 2
Date:
Focus: Endurance

SLEEP   Total Time   _____

            Quality   1   2   3   4   5

MOBILITY

ENDURANCE

	2 miles ruck	35 pounds
Time:	_____	
Run	30 min - Z2	30 min - Z3
Mileage:	_____	_____
Avg HR:	_____	_____

Be fast, but don't worry about speed. Concentrate on technique, stride, misery management, and breathing.

Cognition Prompt: Why are you going to SFAS?
If you had to boil it down to 1 or 2 specific reasons, what would they be?

Conditions   Temperature: _____

              Humidity: _____

          Time of Day: _____

Socks: _____   Boots: _____

Hotspots: _____

NUTRITION   GOAL

        TOTAL CALORIES: _____ _____

   GRAMS OF PROTEIN: _____ _____

           HYDRATION: _____ _____

WEEK 11 - DAY 3
Date:
Focus: Strength

SLEEP   Total Time   _____
             Quality   1   2   3   4   5

MOBILITY

STRENGTH   80% 1RM   3 Sets   10-15 Reps

SQUAT Wt   / Reps Wt   / Reps Wt   / Reps

DEADLIFT Wt   / Reps Wt   / Reps Wt   / Reps

OHP Wt   / Reps Wt   / Reps Wt   / Reps

1-2 minutes rest between sets

NUTRITION   GOAL
        TOTAL CALORIES: _____ _____
      GRAMS OF PROTEIN: _____ _____
             HYDRATION: _____ _____

READING: _____

RESEARCH: _____

WEEK 11 – DAY 4
Date:
Focus: Endurance

SLEEP   Total Time   _____
              Quality   1   2   3   4   5

MOBILITY

ENDURANCE   2 miles ruck   35 pounds
                Time: _____
                       60 min run   Zone 2
             Mileage: _____
              Avg HR: _____

Cognition Prompt: What does the ruck feel like on my back?
How are the straps positioned?
How is the weight distribution?
How does the weight of the ruck change during each step or as I cover different terrain?
How can this information help me refine how I prepare my ruck in the future?

Conditions   Temperature: _____
                  Humidity: _____
               Time of Day: _____

Socks: _____   Boots: _____
Hotspots: _____

NUTRITION   GOAL
        TOTAL CALORIES: _____   _____
      GRAMS OF PROTEIN: _____   _____
             HYDRATION: _____   _____

WEEK 11 - DAY 5
Date:
Focus: Strength

SLEEP   Total Time   _____

Quality   1   2   3   4   5

MOBILITY

STRENGTH   80% 1RM   3 Sets   10-15 Reps

Bench Wt / Reps Wt / Reps Wt / Reps
_____

Row Wt / Reps Wt / Reps Wt / Reps
_____

Shrug Wt / Reps Wt / Reps Wt / Reps
_____

1-2 minutes rest between sets

EMERGING LIMITATIONS: _____

EMERGING CAPABILITIES: _____

NUTRITION   GOAL
TOTAL CALORIES: _____ _____
GRAMS OF PROTEIN: _____ _____
HYDRATION: _____ _____

READING: _____

RESEARCH: _____

WEEK 11 - DAY 6
Date:
Focus: Endurance

SLEEP Total Time _____

Quality   1   2   3   4   5

MOBILITY

ENDURANCE   2 miles ruck   35 pounds

Time: _____

Run   12 x 400 - Z4
1:2 work:rest

Solve this critical thinking question. Answer on bottom of page

What is one thing that these items all have in common?

Jaguar, Falcon, Jet, Bear, Charger

Conditions   Temperature: _____
Humidity: _____
Time of Day: _____

Socks: _____   Boots: _____
Hotspots: _____

NUTRITION   GOAL
TOTAL CALORIES: _____ ____
GRAMS OF PROTEIN: _____ ____
HYDRATION: _____ ____

(all of these are mascots for NFL teams)

WEEK 11 - DAY 7
Date:
Focus: Rest

<u>SLEEP</u>   Total Time   _____

                Quality   1   2   3   4   5

<u>MOBILITY</u>

SUMMARY	SLEEP	CALORIES	PROTEIN	HYDRATION
Day 1				
Day 2				
Day 3				
Day 4				
Day 5				
Day 6				
Day 7				

EMERGING LIMITATIONS: _____

EMERGING CAPABILITIES: _____

<u>NUTRITION</u>   GOAL

            TOTAL CALORIES: _____ _____

        GRAMS OF PROTEIN: _____ _____

                  HYDRATION: _____ _____

NEXT WEEK TRAINING FOCUS: _____

_____

_____

WEEK 12 - SUMMARY

Set patterns. Figure out your ruck set-up, your boots and socks, and your foot care. Be in charge of yourself. You are building resiliency, so be resilient.

DAY 1	MOBILITY 1	STRENGTH WORK
DAY 2	MOBILITY 2	ENDURANCE WORK
DAY 3	MOBILITY 1	STRENGTH WORK
DAY 4	MOBILITY 2	ENDURANCE WORK
DAY 5	MOBILITY 1	STRENGTH WORK
DAY 6	MOBILITY 2	SKILLS WORK
DAY 7		REST

You are taking notes for a reason, use them. Set your skill workout for Day 6 based off of your notes about skills progression, weaknesses, mobility issues, and training goals.

You have 2 rucks with 6 miles this week.

Do you want to be competent and dangerous or vague and useless?

WEEK 12 - DAY 1
Date:
Focus: Strength

SLEEP   Total Time   _____

           Quality   1   2   3   4   5

MOBILITY

STRENGTH   80% 1RM   3 Sets   10-15 Reps

	Wt	/	Reps	Wt	/	Reps	Wt	/	Reps
SQUAT									
DEADLIFT									
OHP									

1-2 minutes rest between sets

EMERGING LIMITATIONS: _____

EMERGING CAPABILITIES: _____

NUTRITION   GOAL

           TOTAL CALORIES: _____ ___

      GRAMS OF PROTEIN: _____ ___

                HYDRATION: _____ ___

READING: _____

RESEARCH: _____

WEEK 12 - DAY 2
Date:
Focus: Endurance

SLEEP   Total Time   _____

Quality   1   2   3   4   5

MOBILITY

ENDURANCE   3 miles ruck   35 pounds

Time: _____

Run   25 min - Z2   20 min - Z3

Mileage: _____   _____

Avg HR: _____   _____

Cognition Prompt: Become aware of your surroundings. Have you run/rucked in this gym/trail/road before? Whether or not you have, reflect on what things in this environment that you have either seen before or are familiar to things you have seen before. What things are unique or novel to your PT today?

Socks: _____   Boots: _____

Hotspots: _____

NUTRITION   GOAL

TOTAL CALORIES: _____ _____

GRAMS OF PROTEIN: _____ _____

HYDRATION: _____ _____

READING: _____

RESEARCH: _____

WEEK 12 - DAY 3
Date:
Focus: Strength

SLEEP   Total Time   _____
                    Quality   1   2   3   4   5

MOBILITY

STRENGTH   80% 1RM   3 Sets   10-15 Reps

Bench   Wt   /   Reps   Wt   /   Reps   Wt   /   Reps
_____

Row   Wt   /   Reps   Wt   /   Reps   Wt   /   Reps
_____

Shrug   Wt   /   Reps   Wt   /   Reps   Wt   /   Reps
_____

1-2 minutes rest between sets

NUTRITION   GOAL
              TOTAL CALORIES: _____ _____
           GRAMS OF PROTEIN: _____ _____
                    HYDRATION: _____ _____

READING: _____

RESEARCH: _____

Date:

Focus: Endurance

SLEEP   Total Time   _____

Quality   1   2   3   4   5

MOBILITY

ENDURANCE   3 miles ruck   35 pounds

Time: _____

45 min run   Zone 2

Mileage: _____

Avg HR: _____

Cognition Prompt: What are your biggest strengths and qualities that you possess?
Which new ones would you prioritize developing?
How often do you allow yourself to lead with your strengths?

Socks: _____   Boots: _____

Hotspots: _____

NUTRITION   GOAL

TOTAL CALORIES: _____ _____

GRAMS OF PROTEIN: _____ _____

HYDRATION: _____ _____

READING: _____

RESEARCH: _____

WEEK 12 - DAY 5
Date:
Focus: Strength

SLEEP   Total Time   _____

              Quality   1   2   3   4   5

MOBILITY

STRENGTH   80% 1RM   3 Sets   10-15 Reps

SQUAT   Wt   /   Reps   Wt   /   Reps   Wt   /   Reps
_____

DEADLIFT   Wt   /   Reps   Wt   /   Reps   Wt   /   Reps
_____

OHP   Wt   /   Reps   Wt   /   Reps   Wt   /   Reps
_____

1-2 minutes rest between sets

EMERGING LIMITATIONS: _____

EMERGING CAPABILITIES: _____

NUTRITION   GOAL
              TOTAL CALORIES: _____   _____
            GRAMS OF PROTEIN: _____   _____
                  HYDRATION: _____   _____

READING: _____

RESEARCH: _____

WEEK 12 - DAY 6
Date:
Focus: Skills

SLEEP   Total Time   _____

                 Quality   1   2   3   4   5

MOBILITY

SKILLS   From Menu

NUTRITION   GOAL

            TOTAL CALORIES: _____ _____

       GRAMS OF PROTEIN: _____ _____

                HYDRATION: _____ _____

READING: _____

RESEARCH: _____

WEEK 12 – DAY 7
Date:
Focus: Rest

SLEEP   Total Time   _____

              Quality   1   2   3   4   5

MOBILITY

SUMMARY	SLEEP	CALORIES	PROTEIN	HYDRATION
Day 1				
Day 2				
Day 3				
Day 4				
Day 5				
Day 6				
Day 7				

EMERGING LIMITATIONS: _____

EMERGING CAPABILITIES: _____

NUTRITION   GOAL
              TOTAL CALORIES: _____ _____
            GRAMS OF PROTEIN: _____ _____
                   HYDRATION: _____ _____

NEXT WEEK TRAINING FOCUS: _____

_____

_____

WEEK 13 - SUMMARY

You will check in on your PFT and FMS progress so that you can continue to refine your warm-up and movement prep. Strength, endurance, skills, and speed. All the rules matter.

DAY 1	MOBILITY 1	ASSESSMENT
DAY 2	MOBILITY 2	ENDURANCE WORK
DAY 3	MOBILITY 1	STRENGTH WORK
DAY 4	MOBILITY 2	ENDURANCE WORK
DAY 5	MOBILITY 1	STRENGTH WORK
DAY 6	MOBILITY 2	SKILLS & SPEED
DAY 7		REST

You have 2 rucks with 6 miles this week.

It's not supposed to be comfortable.

WEEK 13 - DAY 1

Date:

Focus: assessment

SLEEP   Total Time   _____

           Quality   1   2   3   4   5

PFA

HRPU	
PLANK	
PULL-UPS	
2 MILE RUN	

DEEP SQUAT	0	1	2	3
INLINE LUNGE	0	1	2	3
HURDLE STEP	0	1	2	3
SHOULDER MOBILITY	0	1	2	3
ACTIVE STRAIGHT LEG RAISE	0	1	2	3
TRUNK STABILITY PUSH UP	0	1	2	3
ROTATIONAL STABILITY	0	1	2	3

0: You feel any pain at all

1: You can do the move, but not very well

2. You can do the move, but you need to compensate in some way.

3. You can perfectly master the move.

NUTRITION   GOAL

    TOTAL CALORIES: _____ _____

    GRAMS OF PROTEIN: _____ _____

    HYDRATION: _____ _____

READING: _____

RESEARCH: _____

WEEK 13 - DAY 2
Date:
Focus: Endurance

SLEEP   Total Time   _____

Quality   1   2   3   4   5

MOBILITY

ENDURANCE   3 miles ruck   35 pounds

Time: _____

Run   25 min - Z2   20 min - Z3

Mileage: _____   _____

Avg HR: _____   _____

Cognition Prompt (KIMS Game): Commit this list of random items to memory:
1. Candy Wrapper 2. Clay Pot 3. Keys 4. Rubber Duck 5. Piano 6. Spandex   How
many can you remember after the workout?

Socks: _____   Boots: _____

Hotspots: _____

NUTRITION   GOAL

TOTAL CALORIES: _____   _____

GRAMS OF PROTEIN: _____   _____

HYDRATION: _____   _____

READING: _____

RESEARCH: _____

WEEK 13 - DAY 3
Date:
Focus: Strength

SLEEP   Total Time   _____
              Quality   1   2   3   4   5

MOBILITY

STRENGTH   80% 1RM   3 Sets   10-15 Reps

Bench Wt / Reps Wt / Reps Wt / Reps
_____

Row Wt / Reps Wt / Reps Wt / Reps
_____

Shrug Wt / Reps Wt / Reps Wt / Reps
_____

1-2 minutes rest between sets

NUTRITION   GOAL
          TOTAL CALORIES: _____ _____
        GRAMS OF PROTEIN: _____ _____
              HYDRATION: _____ _____

READING: _____

RESEARCH: _____

WEEK 13 - DAY 4
Date:
Focus: Endurance

<u>SLEEP</u>   Total Time _____

                Quality   1   2   3   4   5

<u>MOBILITY</u>

<u>ENDURANCE</u>   3 miles ruck   35 pounds

                Time: _____

                45 min run   Zone 2

         Mileage: _____

         Avg HR: _____

Solve this critical thinking question. Answer at the bottom of the page.
Which is the odd item out? Why?
2, 3, 5, 7, 11, 13, 17, 19, 23, 29, 33, 37

Socks: _____   Boots: _____
Hotspots: _____

<u>NUTRITION</u>   GOAL

        TOTAL CALORIES: _____ _____

      GRAMS OF PROTEIN: _____ _____

             HYDRATION: _____ _____

READING: _____

RESEARCH: _____

33 (All of the rest are prime numbers)

WEEK 13 - DAY 5
Date:
Focus: Strength

SLEEP   Total Time   _____
              Quality   1   2   3   4   5

MOBILITY

STRENGTH   80% 1RM   3 Sets   10-15 Reps

SQUAT   Wt   /   Reps   Wt   /   Reps   Wt   /   Reps

DEADLIFT Wt   /   Reps   Wt   /   Reps   Wt   /   Reps

OHP   Wt   /   Reps   Wt   /   Reps   Wt   /   Reps

1-2 minutes rest between sets

EMERGING LIMITATIONS: _____

EMERGING CAPABILITIES: _____

NUTRITION   GOAL
        TOTAL CALORIES: _____   _____
       GRAMS OF PROTEIN: _____   _____
            HYDRATION: _____   _____

READING: _____

RESEARCH: _____

WEEK 13 - DAY 6
Date:
Focus: Skills and Speed

SLEEP   Total Time   _____

             Quality   1   2   3   4   5

MOBILITY

SKILLS   From Menu

SPEED   12 x 400 - Z4

                  1:2 work:rest

NUTRITION   GOAL

        TOTAL CALORIES: _____ _____

    GRAMS OF PROTEIN: _____ _____

            HYDRATION: _____ _____

READING: _____

RESEARCH: _____

WEEK 13 - DAY 7
Date:
Focus: Rest

SLEEP   Total Time   _____

                Quality   1   2   3   4   5

MOBILITY

SUMMARY	SLEEP	CALORIES	PROTEIN	HYDRATION
Day 1				
Day 2				
Day 3				
Day 4				
Day 5				
Day 6				
Day 7				

EMERGING LIMITATIONS: _____

EMERGING CAPABILITIES: _____

NUTRITION   GOAL

        TOTAL CALORIES: _____ _____

      GRAMS OF PROTEIN: _____ _____

            HYDRATION: _____ _____

NEXT WEEK TRAINING FOCUS: _____

MOBILITY WORKSHEET

MOBILITY WORKSHEET

WEEK 14 - SUMMARY

You should be noticing real changes in your performance at this point. If you aren't seeing significant improvements then you need to evaluate all of this data that you are collecting. Are you sleeping enough? Is it quality sleep? Are you getting enough protein? If your endurance is suffering then are you getting enough carbs? You need carbs, too. How is your hydration. All of this stuff matters.

DAY 1	MOBILITY 1	STRENGTH WORK
DAY 2	MOBILITY 2	ENDURANCE WORK
DAY 3	MOBILITY 1	STRENGTH WORK
DAY 4	MOBILITY 2	ENDURANCE WORK
DAY 5	MOBILITY 1	STRENGTH WORK
DAY 6	MOBILITY 2	ENDURANCE & SPEED
DAY 7		REST

The workouts are easy, its the lifestyle that challenges you.

You have 3 rucks with 9 miles this week and the ruck weight increases.

Make them remember you. Earn your humility.

WEEK 14 - DAY 1
Date:
Focus: Strength

SLEEP   Total Time   _____
             Quality   1   2   3   4   5

MOBILITY

STRENGTH   90% 1RM   4 Sets   8-10 Reps

Bench   Wt / Reps   Wt / Reps   Wt / Reps   Wt / Reps

Row   Wt / Reps   Wt / Reps   Wt / Reps   Wt / Reps

Shrug   Wt / Reps   Wt / Reps   Wt / Reps   Wt / Reps

2-4 minutes rest between sets

EMERGING LIMITATIONS: _____

EMERGING CAPABILITIES: _____

NUTRITION   GOAL
    TOTAL CALORIES: _____   _____
    GRAMS OF PROTEIN: _____   _____
    HYDRATION: _____   _____

READING: _____

RESEARCH: _____

WEEK 14 – DAY 2
Date:
Focus: Endurance

<u>**SLEEP**</u>   Total Time   _____

Quality   1   2   3   4   5

<u>**MOBILITY**</u>

<u>**ENDURANCE**</u>   3 miles ruck   40 pounds

Time: _____

Run   25 min - Z2   20 min - Z3

Mileage: _____   _____

Avg HR: _____   _____

Cognition Prompt: Today you will be prioritizing the different things that you hear in your surroundings. See if you can identify all the various sounds around you. When you identify a sound, allow yourself to label or categorize it, and then broaden your awareness back out to look for more. Try not to get 'stuck' thinking or wondering about any particular sound.

Socks: _____   Boots: _____

Hotspots: _____

<u>**NUTRITION**</u>   GOAL

TOTAL CALORIES: _____ _____

GRAMS OF PROTEIN: _____ _____

HYDRATION: _____ _____

READING: _____

RESEARCH: _____

WEEK 14 - DAY 3

Date:

Focus: Strength

SLEEP   Total Time   _____

Quality   1   2   3   4   5

MOBILITY

STRENGTH   80% 1RM   3 Sets   10-15 Reps

SQUAT   Wt / Reps   Wt / Reps   Wt / Reps

DEADLIFT   Wt / Reps   Wt / Reps   Wt / Reps

OHP   Wt / Reps   Wt / Reps   Wt / Reps

1-2 minutes rest between sets

NUTRITION   GOAL

TOTAL CALORIES: _____   _____

GRAMS OF PROTEIN: _____   _____

HYDRATION: _____   _____

READING: _____

RESEARCH: _____

SLEEP   Total Time   _____

Quality   1   2   3   4   5

MOBILITY

ENDURANCE   3 miles ruck   40 pounds

Time: _____

45 min run   Zone 2

Mileage: _____

Avg HR: _____

Cognition Prompt: If you could read the mind of the people closest to you, what would you hope their thoughts about you would look like?

Socks: _____   Boots: _____

Hotspots: _____

NUTRITION   GOAL

TOTAL CALORIES: _____ _____

GRAMS OF PROTEIN: _____ _____

HYDRATION: _____ _____

READING: _____

RESEARCH: _____

WEEK 14 - DAY 5
Date:
Focus: Strength

SLEEP   Total Time   _____

             Quality   1   2   3   4   5

MOBILITY

STRENGTH   80% 1RM   3 Sets   10-15 Reps

Bench Wt / Reps Wt / Reps Wt / Reps

Row Wt / Reps Wt / Reps Wt / Reps

Shrug Wt / Reps Wt / Reps Wt / Reps

1-2 minutes rest between sets

EMERGING LIMITATIONS: _____

EMERGING CAPABILITIES: _____

NUTRITION   GOAL

        TOTAL CALORIES: _____ _____

     GRAMS OF PROTEIN: _____ _____

            HYDRATION: _____ _____

READING: _____

RESEARCH: _____

WEEK 14 - DAY 6
Date:
Focus: Endurance

SLEEP　　Total Time　　_____

Quality　　　1　　2　　3　　4　　5

MOBILITY

ENDURANCE　　　　3 miles ruck　　40 pounds

Time:　_____

SPEED　　　　　Run　　　8 x 400 - Z4

1:2 work:rest

Cognition Prompt (KIMS Game): Commit this list of random items to memory.
1. Lamp Shade 2. Cup 3. Radio 4. Camera 5. Sticky Note 6. Ice cube 7. Bottle　　How many can you remember after the workout?

Socks: _____　　Boots: _____

Hotspots: _____

NUTRITION　　　　　　　　　　　　　　GOAL

TOTAL CALORIES: _____ _____

GRAMS OF PROTEIN: _____ _____

HYDRATION: _____ _____

READING: _____

RESEARCH: _____

WEEK 14 - DAY 7
Date:
Focus: Rest

SLEEP Total Time _____

Quality 1   2   3   4   5

MOBILITY

SUMMARY	SLEEP	CALORIES	PROTEIN	HYDRATION
Day 1				
Day 2				
Day 3				
Day 4				
Day 5				
Day 6				
Day 7				

EMERGING LIMITATIONS: _____

EMERGING CAPABILITIES: _____

NUTRITION   GOAL

TOTAL CALORIES: _____ _____

GRAMS OF PROTEIN: _____ _____

HYDRATION: _____ _____

NEXT WEEK TRAINING FOCUS: _____

WEEK 15 - SUMMARY

We are jumping our strength progression to 90% this week for the next 2 weeks. You're ready.

DAY 1	MOBILITY 1	STRENGTH WORK
DAY 2	MOBILITY 2	ENDURANCE WORK
DAY 3	MOBILITY 1	STRENGTH WORK
DAY 4	MOBILITY 2	ENDURANCE WORK
DAY 5	MOBILITY 1	STRENGTH WORK
DAY 6	MOBILITY 2	SKILLS & SPEED
DAY 7		REST

You have 2 rucks with 8 miles this week.

If you can't be dependable for yourself, how can your teammates trust you?

WEEK 15 - DAY 1
Date:
Focus: Strength

SLEEP   Total Time   _____
             Quality   1   2   3   4   5

MOBILITY

STRENGTH   90% 1RM   4 Sets   8-10 Reps

Squat	Wt	/	Reps	Wt	/	Reps	Wt	/	Reps	Wt	/	Reps

Deadlift	Wt	/	Reps	Wt	/	Reps	Wt	/	Reps	Wt	/	Reps

OHP	Wt	/	Reps	Wt	/	Reps	Wt	/	Reps	Wt	/	Reps

2-4 minutes rest between sets

EMERGING LIMITATIONS: _____

EMERGING CAPABILITIES: _____

NUTRITION   GOAL
           TOTAL CALORIES: _____
       GRAMS OF PROTEIN: _____
              HYDRATION: _____

READING: _____

RESEARCH: _____

Date:

Focus: Endurance

SLEEP   Total Time   _____

              Quality   1   2   3   4   5

MOBILITY

ENDURANCE   4 miles ruck   40 pounds

                    Time: _____

                          30 min run - Z2

              Mileage: _____

              Avg HR: _____

Cognition Prompt: Solve this critical thinking question. Answer at the bottom of the page.
A man is looking at a photograph of someone. His friend asks who it is. The man replies,
"Brothers and sisters, I have none. But that man's father is my father's son." Who was in the
photograph?

Socks: _____   Boots: _____

Hotspots: _____

NUTRITION   GOAL

              TOTAL CALORIES: _____ _____

              GRAMS OF PROTEIN: _____ _____

              HYDRATION: _____ _____

READING: _____

RESEARCH: _____

Answer: His Son

WEEK 15 - DAY 3

Date:

Focus: Strength

SLEEP   Total Time   _____

Quality   1   2   3   4   5

MOBILITY

STRENGTH   90% 1RM   4 Sets   8-10 Reps

Bench   Wt   /   Reps   Wt   /   Reps   Wt   /   Reps   Wt   /   Reps

Row   Wt   /   Reps   Wt   /   Reps   Wt   /   Reps   Wt   /   Reps

Shrug   Wt   /   Reps   Wt   /   Reps   Wt   /   Reps   Wt   /   Reps

2-4 minutes rest between sets

NUTRITION   GOAL

TOTAL CALORIES: _____   _____

GRAMS OF PROTEIN: _____   _____

HYDRATION: _____   _____

READING: _____

RESEARCH: _____

WEEK 15 – DAY 4
Date:
Focus: Endurance

SLEEP   Total Time   _____

             Quality   1   2   3   4   5

MOBILITY

ENDURANCE   4 miles ruck   40 pounds

                   Time: _____

                          30 min run   Zone 2

             Mileage: _____

             Avg HR: _____

Cognition Prompt: Focus on how you are changing the environment around you. How much noise or sound is being generated by you alone? What evidence of your presence is left behind in this space? Are you disturbing, in any way, the natural manner of things? Can you minimize your impact by becoming consciously aware of it?

Socks: _____   Boots: _____

Hotspots: _____

NUTRITION   GOAL

         TOTAL CALORIES: _____ _____

     GRAMS OF PROTEIN: _____ _____

             HYDRATION: _____ _____

READING: _____

RESEARCH: _____

WEEK 15 - DAY 5
Date:
Focus: Strength

SLEEP   Total Time   _____

Quality   1   2   3   4   5

MOBILITY

STRENGTH   90% 1RM   4 Sets   8-10 Reps

	Wt	/	Reps	Wt	/	Reps	Wt	/	Reps	Wt	/	Reps
Squat												
Deadlift												
OHP												

2-4 minutes rest between sets

EMERGING LIMITATIONS: _____

EMERGING CAPABILITIES: _____

NUTRITION   GOAL

TOTAL CALORIES: _____ _____

GRAMS OF PROTEIN: _____ _____

HYDRATION: _____ _____

READING: _____

RESEARCH: _____

WEEK 15 – DAY 6
Date:
Focus: Skills & Speed

SLEEP   Total Time   _____
               Quality   1   2   3   4   5

MOBILITY

SKILLS   From Menu

SPEED   Run   10 x 400 – Z4
                                  1:2 work:rest

NUTRITION   GOAL
        TOTAL CALORIES: _____ _____
    GRAMS OF PROTEIN: _____ _____
            HYDRATION: _____ _____

READING: _____

RESEARCH: _____

WEEK 15 - DAY 7
Date:
Focus: Rest

SLEEP   Total Time   _____

Quality   1   2   3   4   5

MOBILITY

SUMMARY	SLEEP	CALORIES	PROTEIN	HYDRATION
Day 1				
Day 2				
Day 3				
Day 4				
Day 5				
Day 6				
Day 7				

EMERGING LIMITATIONS: _____

EMERGING CAPABILITIES: _____

NUTRITION   GOAL

TOTAL CALORIES: _____ _____

GRAMS OF PROTEIN: _____ _____

HYDRATION: _____ _____

NEXT WEEK TRAINING FOCUS: _____

_____

_____

WEEK 16 - SUMMARY

Lots of running and rucking volume this week. Be cognizant of your recovery, sleep, and nutrition.

DAY 1	MOBILITY 1	STRENGTH WORK
DAY 2	MOBILITY 2	ENDURANCE WORK
DAY 3	MOBILITY 1	STRENGTH WORK
DAY 4	MOBILITY 2	ENDURANCE WORK
DAY 5	MOBILITY 1	STRENGTH WORK
DAY 6	MOBILITY 2	ENDURANCE & SPEED
DAY 7		REST

You have 3 rucks with 12 miles this week.

Pressure is a privilege.

Date:

Focus: Strength

SLEEP   Total Time   _____

Quality   1   2   3   4   5

MOBILITY

STRENGTH   90% 1RM   4 Sets   8-10 Reps

Bench   Wt / Reps   Wt / Reps   Wt / Reps   Wt / Reps

Row   Wt / Reps   Wt / Reps   Wt / Reps   Wt / Reps

Shrug   Wt / Reps   Wt / Reps   Wt / Reps   Wt / Reps

2-4 minutes rest between sets

EMERGING LIMITATIONS: _____

EMERGING CAPABILITIES: _____

NUTRITION   GOAL

TOTAL CALORIES: _____   _____

GRAMS OF PROTEIN: _____   _____

HYDRATION: _____   _____

READING: _____

RESEARCH: _____

WEEK 16 - DAY 2
Date:
Focus: Endurance

SLEEP   Total Time   _____

Quality   1   2   3   4   5

MOBILITY

ENDURANCE   4 miles ruck   40 pounds

Time: _____

Run   25 min - Z2   20 min - Z3

Mileage: _____   _____

Avg HR:

Cognition Prompt: What are examples from your life in which you failed to reach your expectations?
What can you learn from those situations in order to make sure it doesn't happen this time around?

Socks: _____   Boots: _____

Hotspots: _____

NUTRITION   GOAL

TOTAL CALORIES: _____   _____

GRAMS OF PROTEIN: _____   _____

HYDRATION: _____   _____

READING: _____

RESEARCH: _____

WEEK 16 - DAY 3
Date:
Focus: Strength

SLEEP   Total Time   _____

             Quality   1   2   3   4   5

MOBILITY

STRENGTH   90% 1RM   4 Sets   8-10 Reps

	Wt	/	Reps	Wt	/	Reps	Wt	/	Reps	Wt	/	Reps
Squat												
Deadlift												
OHP												

2-4 minutes rest between sets

NUTRITION   GOAL

          TOTAL CALORIES: _____ _____

     GRAMS OF PROTEIN: _____ _____

             HYDRATION: _____ _____

READING: _____

RESEARCH: _____

<u>SLEEP</u> Total Time _____
Quality   1   2   3   4   5

<u>MOBILITY</u>

<u>ENDURANCE</u>   4 miles ruck   40 pounds
Time: _____
45 min run   Zone 2
Mileage: _____
Avg HR: _____

Cognition Prompt: Complete this creativity exercise.

Choose a random object. It can really be anything, such as a paper clip. Aim to generate as many possible uses for this object as you can.

Socks: _____   Boots: _____
Hotspots: _____

<u>NUTRITION</u>   GOAL
TOTAL CALORIES: _____ _____
GRAMS OF PROTEIN: _____ _____
HYDRATION: _____ _____

READING: _____

RESEARCH: _____

WEEK 16 - DAY 5
Date:
Focus: Strength

SLEEP   Total Time   _____

Quality   1   2   3   4   5

MOBILITY

STRENGTH   90% 1RM   4 Sets   8-10 Reps

Bench   Wt / Reps   Wt / Reps   Wt / Reps   Wt / Reps

Row   Wt / Reps   Wt / Reps   Wt / Reps   Wt / Reps

Shrug   Wt / Reps   Wt / Reps   Wt   Reps   Wt / Reps

2-4 minutes rest between sets

EMERGING LIMITATIONS: _____

EMERGING CAPABILITIES: _____

NUTRITION   GOAL

TOTAL CALORIES: _____ _____

GRAMS OF PROTEIN: _____ _____

HYDRATION: _____ _____

READING: _____

RESEARCH: _____

WEEK 16 - DAY 6
Date:
Focus: Endurance and Speed

SLEEP   Total Time   _____

             Quality   1   2   3   4   5

MOBILITY

ENDURANCE   4 miles ruck   40 pounds

                Time: _____

SPEED   Run   10 x 400 - Z4

                          1:2 work:rest

Cognition Prompt (KIMS Game): Commit this list of random items to memory.

1. Pool Cue 2. Controller 3. Cork 4. Needle 5. Ring 6. Toothpaste 7. Charger 8. Magnet

---

Socks: _____   Boots: _____

Hotspots: _____

NUTRITION   GOAL

        TOTAL CALORIES: _____ _____

        GRAMS OF PROTEIN: _____ _____

              HYDRATION: _____ _____

READING: _____

RESEARCH: _____

WEEK 16 – DAY 7
Date:
Focus: Rest

SLEEP   Total Time   _____

            Quality   1   2   3   4   5

MOBILITY

SUMMARY	SLEEP	CALORIES	PROTEIN	HYDRATION
Day 1				
Day 2				
Day 3				
Day 4				
Day 5				
Day 6				
Day 7				

EMERGING LIMITATIONS: _____

EMERGING CAPABILITIES: _____

NUTRITION   GOAL

        TOTAL CALORIES: _____ _____

      GRAMS OF PROTEIN: _____ _____

            HYDRATION: _____ _____

NEXT WEEK TRAINING FOCUS: _____

WEEK 17 - SUMMARY

   This week we test out of Phase 2 and start Phase 3 and it is all about re-establishing baseline metrics across all of the domains that we have been training so that we can see how far we have come...and decide if we are ready to proceed with this next phase or re-engage for a few weeks to meet the prerequisites. If you are unable to 1RM Bench Press 1x your BW, 1.5x BW 1RM Squat, and 1.75x BW 1RM Deadlift then you are not ready to proceed. Repeat the last 4 weeks. This program is not time driven, it is performance driven. Do not rush to failure.

DAY 1	FMS	Functional Movement Screening
DAY 2	PFA	Physical Fitness Assessment
DAY 3	1RM	1 Repetition Maximum Lift
DAY 4	5 MILE RUN	5 Mile Run
DAY 5	RUCK	12 Mile Ruck Assessment
DAY 6	REST	Rest, Journal, Plan, Meal Prep
DAY 7	REST	Rest, Journal, Plan, Meal Prep

The data does not lie. You are 4 months into program. You should have made significant progress in every domain. The programming is solid, so if you are not making significant progress then you either need to see a medical professional for an evaluation, or you need to get your diet, sleep, hydration, and recovery in order. The program is simply stimuli that the body must adapt to.

Nothing can resist the human will that stakes even its existence on its stated purpose.

- Benjamin Disraeli

WEEK 17 - DAY 1
Date:
Focus: Functional Movement Screening

SLEEP   Total Time _____

             Quality   1   2   3   4   5

DEEP SQUAT	0	1	2 3
INLINE LUNGE	0	1	2 3
HURDLE STEP	0	1	2 3
SHOULDER MOBILITY	0	1	2 3
ACTIVE STRAIGHT LEG RAISE	0	1	2 3
TRUNK STABILITY PUSH UP	0	1	2 3
ROTATIONAL STABILITY	0	1	2 3

0: You feel any pain at all

1: You can do the move, but not very well

2. You can do the move, but you need to compensate in some way.

3. You can perfectly master the move.

Height: _____
Weight: _____

NUTRITION   GOAL

       TOTAL CALORIES: _____ _____

   GRAMS OF PROTEIN: _____ _____

           HYDRATION: _____ _____

READING: _____

RESEARCH: _____

WEEK 17 - DAY 2
Date:
Focus: PHYSICAL FITNESS ASSESSMENT

SLEEP   Total Time _____

Quality   1   2   3   4   5

PFA

HRPU	
PLANK	
PULL-UPS	
2 MILE RUN	

NUTRITION   GOAL

TOTAL CALORIES: _____ _____

GRAMS OF PROTEIN: _____ _____

HYDRATION: _____ _____

READING: _____

RESEARCH: _____

WEEK 17 - DAY 3
Date:
Focus: ESTABLISH 1 REP MAX

SLEEP   Total Time   _____
              Quality   1   2   3   4   5

MOBILITY

STRENGTH

                    SQUAT   _____

                 DEADLIFT   _____

                    BENCH   _____

                      ROW   _____

                    SHRUG   _____

                      OHP   _____

NUTRITION   GOAL
          TOTAL CALORIES: _____ _____
        GRAMS OF PROTEIN: _____ _____
              HYDRATION: _____ _____

READING: _____

RESEARCH: _____

<u>SLEEP</u>   Total Time   _____

             Quality   1   2   3   4   5

<u>MOBILITY</u>

<u>5 MILE RUN</u>

                  TIME   _____

         AVERAGE HR: _____

         <u>Conditions</u>

           Temperature: _____

              Humidity: _____

            Time of Day: _____

SHOES   _____

SOCKS   _____

HOT SPOTS _____

PAIN POINTS _____

<u>NUTRITION</u>   GOAL

        TOTAL CALORIES: _____ _____

     GRAMS OF PROTEIN: _____ _____

           HYDRATION: _____ _____

READING: _____

RESEARCH: _____

SLEEP   Total Time _____

           Quality   1   2   3   4   5

RUCK   12 miles   40 pounds

              TIME _____

     AVERAGE HR: _____

          Conditions

        Temperature: _____

          Humidity: _____

       Time of Day: _____

BOOTS _____

SOCKS _____

HOT SPOTS _____

PAIN POINTS _____

NUTRITION   GOAL

     TOTAL CALORIES: _____ _____

  GRAMS OF PROTEIN: _____ _____

         HYDRATION: _____ _____

READING: _____

RESEARCH: _____

WEEK 17 - DAY 6
Date:
Focus: REST

SLEEP   Total Time   _____

Quality   1   2   3   4   5

MOBILITY

Spend some time today redeveloping your mobility, warm-up, and movement prep routines. With the introduction of rucking, you may note some additional requirements.

NUTRITION   GOAL

TOTAL CALORIES: _____ _____

GRAMS OF PROTEIN: _____ _____

HYDRATION: _____ _____

WEEK 17 - DAY 7
Date:
Focus: Rest

SLEEP   Total Time _____
Quality   1   2   3   4   5

MOBILITY

SUMMARY	SLEEP	CALORIES	PROTEIN	HYDRATION
Day 1				
Day 2				
Day 3				
Day 4				
Day 5				
Day 6				
Day 7				

EMERGING LIMITATIONS: _____

EMERGING CAPABILITIES: _____

NUTRITION   GOAL
TOTAL CALORIES: _____ _____
GRAMS OF PROTEIN: _____ _____
HYDRATION: _____ _____

NEXT WEEK TRAINING FOCUS: _____

MOBILITY WORKSHEET

MOBILITY WORKSHEET

WEEK 18 - SUMMARY

Phase 3 Begins. This will also serve as a deload week. You have new 1RM to calculate. We will begin the 5x5 protocol, starting with low mileage and building. Do your squats full range of motion; ass to ankles, hips fully open at the top. We are removing the emerging limitation and capabilities prompts. Go to work.

DAY 1	MOBILITY 1	STRENGTH WORK
DAY 2	MOBILITY 2	ENDURANCE WORK
DAY 3	MOBILITY 1	STRENGTH WORK
DAY 4	MOBILITY 2	ENDURANCE WORK
DAY 5	MOBILITY 1	STRENGTH WORK
DAY 6	MOBILITY 2	SKILLS WORK
DAY 7		REST

You are at about the halfway mark on this program.

Stop telling yourself that you're doing enough. Follow the plan.

WEEK 18 - DAY 1
Date:
Focus: Strength

SLEEP   Total Time   _____

               Quality   1   2   3   4   5

MOBILITY

STRENGTH   80% 1RM   3 Sets   10-15 Reps

SQUAT Wt / Reps   Wt / Reps   Wt / Reps

DEADLIFT Wt / Reps   Wt / Reps   Wt / Reps

OHP Wt / Reps   Wt / Reps   Wt / Reps

1-2 minutes rest between sets

NUTRITION   GOAL

        TOTAL CALORIES: _____ _____

    GRAMS OF PROTEIN: _____ _____

            HYDRATION: _____ _____

READING: _____

RESEARCH: _____

WEEK 18 - DAY 2
Date:
Focus: Endurance

SLEEP   Total Time   _____
          Quality   1   2   3   4   5

MOBILITY

ENDURANCE - 2x2   2 mile ruck   45 pounds
                  Time: _____
                       100 Squats   with ruck
          Run   2 mile run
                  Time: _____
                       100 Squats   without ruck

Cognition Prompt: Complete this creativity exercise.

Identify an object, word, thing, that you encounter. Come up with a story all about this particular item. The story can take whatever direction or turn that you want. There are no limits.

Socks: _____   Boots: _____
Hotspots: _____

NUTRITION   GOAL
          TOTAL CALORIES: _____ _____
          GRAMS OF PROTEIN: _____ _____
          HYDRATION: _____ _____

READING: _____

RESEARCH: _____

SLEEP   Total Time   _____

              Quality   1   2   3   4   5

MOBILITY

STRENGTH   80% 1RM   3 Sets   10-15 Reps

Bench Wt / Reps Wt / Reps Wt / Reps

Row Wt / Reps Wt / Reps Wt / Reps

Shrug Wt / Reps Wt / Reps Wt / Reps

1-2 minutes rest between sets

NUTRITION   GOAL

    TOTAL CALORIES: _____ ____

    GRAMS OF PROTEIN: _____ ____

    HYDRATION: _____ ____

READING: _____

RESEARCH: _____

SLEEP

Total Time _____

Quality   1   2   3   4   5

MOBILITY

ENDURANCE - 2x2

	2 mile ruck	45 pounds
Time: _____		
	100 Squats	with ruck
Run	2 mile run	
Time: _____		
	100 Squats	without ruck

Cognition Prompt: Maintain a soft focus on a short distance in front of you. As you move in the environment, recognize how the visual scene changes, but do so in a way that maintains this soft focus. When your eye sharpens around specific details or features, acknowledge it but bring it back to that soft focus.

Socks: _____   Boots: _____

Hotspots: _____

NUTRITION   GOAL

TOTAL CALORIES: _____ _____

GRAMS OF PROTEIN: _____ _____

HYDRATION: _____ _____

READING: _____

RESEARCH: _____

SLEEP   Total Time _____
              Quality   1   2   3   4   5

MOBILITY

STRENGTH   80% 1RM   3 Sets   10-15 Reps

SQUAT   Wt   /   Reps   Wt   /   Reps   Wt   /   Reps
_____

DEADLIFT Wt   /   Reps   Wt   /   Reps   Wt   /   Reps
_____

OHP   Wt   /   Reps   Wt   /   Reps   Wt   /   Reps
_____

1-2 minutes rest between sets

NUTRITION   GOAL
          TOTAL CALORIES: _____ _____
        GRAMS OF PROTEIN: _____ _____
               HYDRATION: _____ _____

READING: _____

RESEARCH: _____

SLEEP   Total Time   _____

            Quality   1   2   3   4   5

MOBILITY

SKILLS   From Menu

NUTRITION   GOAL

      TOTAL CALORIES: _____ _____

    GRAMS OF PROTEIN: _____ _____

          HYDRATION: _____ _____

READING: _____

RESEARCH: _____

WEEK 18 - DAY 7
Date:
Focus: Rest

SLEEP   Total Time   _____

              Quality   1   2   3   4   5

MOBILITY

SUMMARY	SLEEP	CALORIES	PROTEIN	HYDRATION
Day 1				
Day 2				
Day 3				
Day 4				
Day 5				
Day 6				
Day 7				

NUTRITION   GOAL

            TOTAL CALORIES: _____   _____

         GRAMS OF PROTEIN: _____   _____

                 HYDRATION: _____   _____

NEXT WEEK TRAINING FOCUS: _____

WEEK 19 - SUMMARY

Same as last week, but were adding a speed workout and little Zone 2 session. I warned you that Coach Dave was a freak. But remember that you asked for this, there is no other place you should rather wish to be.

DAY 1	MOBILITY 1	STRENGTH WORK
DAY 2	MOBILITY 2	ENDURANCE WORK
DAY 3	MOBILITY 1	STRENGTH & ENDURANCE
DAY 4	MOBILITY 2	ENDURANCE WORK
DAY 5	MOBILITY 1	STRENGTH & SPEED
DAY 6	MOBILITY 2	ENDURANCE WORK
DAY 7		REST

A man with weak legs is a man with a weak mind.

Date:

Focus: Strength

SLEEP　　Total Time　　_____

　　　　　　Quality　　　　1　　2　　3　　4　　5

MOBILITY

STRENGTH　　80% 1RM　　　3 Sets　　　10-15 Reps

Bench　Wt　/　Reps　Wt　/　Reps　Wt　/　Reps

Row　Wt　/　Reps　Wt　/　Reps　Wt　/　Reps

Shrug　Wt　/　Reps　Wt　/　Reps　Wt　/　Reps

1-2 minutes rest between sets

NUTRITION　　　　　　　　　　　　　　　　　　GOAL

　　　　TOTAL CALORIES: _____ _____

　　GRAMS OF PROTEIN: _____ _____

　　　　　　HYDRATION: _____ _____

READING: _____

RESEARCH: _____

WEEK 19 – DAY 2
Date:
Focus: Endurance

SLEEP   Total Time   _____
           Quality   1   2   3   4   5

MOBILITY

ENDURANCE - 2x2   2 mile ruck   45 pounds
                  Time: _____
                            100 Squats   with ruck
           Run   2 mile run
                  Time: _____
                            100 Squats   without ruck

Cognition Prompt: Who is someone you look up to or hold as a role model?
What are the characteristics that they have that inspire you?

Socks: _____   Boots: _____
Hotspots: _____

NUTRITION   GOAL
           TOTAL CALORIES: _____ _____
          GRAMS OF PROTEIN: _____ _____
               HYDRATION: _____ _____

READING: _____

RESEARCH: _____

WEEK 19 - DAY 3
Date:
Focus: Strength and Endurance

SLEEP   Total Time   _____

              Quality   1   2   3   4   5

MOBILITY

STRENGTH   80% 1RM   3 Sets   10-15 Reps

SQUAT Wt / Reps Wt / Reps Wt / Reps

DEADLIFT Wt / Reps Wt / Reps Wt / Reps

OHP Wt / Reps Wt / Reps Wt / Reps

1-2 minutes rest between sets

ENDURANCE   60 min run   Zone 2

              Mileage: _____

              Avg HR: _____

NUTRITION   GOAL

        TOTAL CALORIES: _____ _____

    GRAMS OF PROTEIN: _____ _____

            HYDRATION: _____ _____

READING: _____

RESEARCH: _____

WEEK 19 - DAY 4
Date:
Focus: Endurance

SLEEP   Total Time   _____

Quality   1   2   3   4   5

MOBILITY

ENDURANCE - 2x2   2 mile ruck   45 pounds

Time: _____

100 Squats   with ruck

Run   2 mile run

Time: _____

100 Squats   without ruck

Cognition Prompt (KIMS Game): Commit this list of random items to memory.

1. Watch 2. Credit Card 3. Milk 4. Lotion 5. Tower 6. Pocket Knife 7. Wheel 8. Bolt 9. Sock

---

Socks: _____   Boots: _____

Hotspots: _____

NUTRITION   GOAL

TOTAL CALORIES: _____ _____

GRAMS OF PROTEIN: _____ _____

HYDRATION: _____ _____

READING: _____

RESEARCH: _____

WEEK 19 - DAY 5
Date:
Focus: Strength & Speed

SLEEP   Total Time   _____
              Quality   1   2   3   4   5

MOBILITY

STRENGTH   80% 1RM   3 Sets   10-15 Reps

	Wt	/	Reps	Wt	/	Reps	Wt	/	Reps
Bench									
Row									
Shrug									

1-2 minutes rest between sets

SPEED   Run   8 x 400 - Z4
                                      1:2 work:rest

NUTRITION   GOAL

        TOTAL CALORIES: _____ _____

    GRAMS OF PROTEIN: _____ _____

           HYDRATION: _____ _____

READING: _____

RESEARCH: _____

WEEK 19 - DAY 6
Date:
Focus: Endurance

SLEEP   Total Time   _____

Quality   1   2   3   4   5

MOBILITY

ENDURANCE - 2x2   2 mile ruck   45 pounds

Time: _____

100 Squats   with ruck

Run   2 mile run

Time: _____

100 Squats   without ruck

Cognition Prompt: Complete this creativity exercise.

What is one problem that you continue to experience that you would love to solve? Identify and develop the concept of a tool that would allow you to solve this problem? What features would it include? What would this tool look like?

Socks: _____   Boots: _____

Hotspots: _____

NUTRITION   GOAL

TOTAL CALORIES: _____ _____

GRAMS OF PROTEIN: _____ _____

HYDRATION: _____ _____

READING: _____

RESEARCH: _____

WEEK 19 - DAY 7
Date:
Focus: Rest

SLEEP   Total Time   _____

                Quality   1   2   3   4   5

MOBILITY

SUMMARY	SLEEP	CALORIES	PROTEIN	HYDRATION
Day 1				
Day 2				
Day 3				
Day 4				
Day 5				
Day 6				
Day 7				

NUTRITION   GOAL

               TOTAL CALORIES: _____ _____

          GRAMS OF PROTEIN: _____ _____

                    HYDRATION: _____ _____

NEXT WEEK TRAINING FOCUS: _____

_____

_____

WEEK 20 - SUMMARY

Only 2 rucks this week, but were adding a mile to each run and we have more speed work. We have another skills day so you should be really refining your skills work. You have the menu of 30 items, but you can add things that you want to work as well.

DAY 1	MOBILITY 1	STRENGTH WORK
DAY 2	MOBILITY 2	ENDURANCE WORK
DAY 3	MOBILITY 1	STRENGTH & ENDURANCE
DAY 4	MOBILITY 2	ENDURANCE WORK
DAY 5	MOBILITY 1	STRENGTH & SPEED
DAY 6	MOBILITY 2	SKILLS WORK
DAY 7		REST

Who is going to stop you?

WEEK 20 - DAY 1
Date:
Focus: Strength

SLEEP   Total Time   _____
             Quality   1   2   3   4   5

MOBILITY

STRENGTH   80% 1RM   3 Sets   10-15 Reps

SQUAT   Wt   /   Reps   Wt   /   Reps   Wt   /   Reps
_____

DEADLIFT   Wt   /   Reps   Wt   /   Reps   Wt   /   Reps
_____

OHP   Wt   /   Reps   Wt   /   Reps   Wt   /   Reps
_____

1-2 minutes rest between sets

NUTRITION   GOAL
             TOTAL CALORIES: _____   _____
         GRAMS OF PROTEIN: _____   _____
                HYDRATION: _____   _____

READING: _____

RESEARCH: _____

SLEEP   Total Time   _____
          Quality   1   2   3   4   5

MOBILITY

ENDURANCE - 2x3   2 mile ruck   45 pounds
          Time: _____
                100 Squats   with ruck
      Run   3 mile run
          Time: _____
                100 Squats   without ruck

Cognition Prompt: Identify the fluctuations of the ground or surface you are moving upon. How do changes in your weight distribution or balance inform you about the terrain? As your body moves, it is directly interacting with the greater environment. Each subtle movement, and your proprioceptive awareness, feed information to you. Study your body as it moves through space. This is especially important when moving under load.

Socks: _____   Boots: _____
Hotspots: _____

NUTRITION   GOAL
      TOTAL CALORIES: _____ _____
   GRAMS OF PROTEIN: _____ _____
         HYDRATION: _____ _____

READING: _____

RESEARCH: _____

WEEK 20 - DAY 3
Date:
Focus: Strength and Endurance

SLEEP   Total Time _____

               Quality   1   2   3   4   5

MOBILITY

STRENGTH   80% 1RM   3 Sets   10-15 Reps

	Wt	/	Reps	Wt	/	Reps	Wt	/	Reps
Bench									
Row									
Shrug									

1-2 minutes rest between sets

ENDURANCE   60 min run   Zone 2

             Mileage: _____

             Avg HR: _____

NUTRITION   GOAL

        TOTAL CALORIES: _____ _____

    GRAMS OF PROTEIN: _____ _____

           HYDRATION: _____ _____

READING: _____

RESEARCH: _____

WEEK 20 - DAY 4
Date:
Focus: Endurance

__SLEEP__   Total Time   _____

                Quality   1   2   3   4   5

__MOBILITY__

__ENDURANCE - 2x3__   2 mile ruck   45 pounds

                 Time: _____

                     100 Squats   with ruck

             Run   3 mile run

                 Time: _____

                     100 Squats   without ruck

Cognition Prompt: Reflect on what you are doing in this 2x3.
How is this choice helping you get closer to your goals, but also move more in alignment to who you strive to be?

Socks: _____   Boots: _____

Hotspots: _____

__NUTRITION__   GOAL

           TOTAL CALORIES: _____ _____

      GRAMS OF PROTEIN: _____ _____

                HYDRATION: _____ _____

READING: _____

RESEARCH: _____

WEEK 20 - DAY 5
Date:
Focus: Strength

SLEEP   Total Time   _____

          Quality   1   2   3   4   5

MOBILITY

STRENGTH   80% 1RM   3 Sets   10-15 Reps

SQUAT Wt / Reps Wt / Reps Wt / Reps

DEADLIFT Wt / Reps Wt / Reps Wt / Reps

OHP Wt / Reps Wt / Reps Wt / Reps

1-2 minutes rest between sets

SPEED   Run   8 x 400 - Z4
                                     1:2 work:rest

NUTRITION   GOAL
          TOTAL CALORIES: _____ _____
          GRAMS OF PROTEIN: _____ _____
          HYDRATION: _____ _____

READING: _____

RESEARCH: _____

SLEEP   Total Time   _____

             Quality   1   2   3   4   5

MOBILITY

SKILLS   From Menu

NUTRITION   GOAL

        TOTAL CALORIES: _____ _____

      GRAMS OF PROTEIN: _____ _____

           HYDRATION: _____ _____

READING: _____

RESEARCH: _____

WEEK 20 - DAY 7
Date:
Focus: Rest

SLEEP   Total Time   _____
Quality   1   2   3   4   5

MOBILITY

SUMMARY	SLEEP	CALORIES	PROTEIN	HYDRATION
Day 1				
Day 2				
Day 3				
Day 4				
Day 5				
Day 6				
Day 7				

NUTRITION   GOAL
TOTAL CALORIES: _____ _____
GRAMS OF PROTEIN: _____ _____
HYDRATION: _____ _____

NEXT WEEK TRAINING FOCUS: _____
_____

WEEK 21 - SUMMARY

A quick assessment on day 1, then right to work. These frequent PFT and FMS assessments should be serving two purposes. First, they give you data to modify and update your warm-up, mobility, and movement prep routines. Second, they should be telling you that a PFT is nothing. It's not some traumatic event. It's the easiest workout that you will do in any given week. You should be crushing them.

DAY 1	MOBILITY 1	ASSESSMENT
DAY 2	MOBILITY 2	ENDURANCE WORK
DAY 3	MOBILITY 1	STRENGTH & ENDURANCE
DAY 4	MOBILITY 2	ENDURANCE WORK
DAY 5	MOBILITY 1	STRENGTH WORK
DAY 6	MOBILITY 2	SKILLS WORK
DAY 7		REST

You might not notice your progress, because you're constantly raising the bar.

WEEK 21 - DAY 1

Date: _____

Focus: Assessment

SLEEP   Total Time   _____

Quality   1   2   3   4   5

PFA

HRPU	
PLANK	
PULL-UPS	
2 MILE RUN	

DEEP SQUAT	0	1	2	3
INLINE LUNGE	0	1	2	3
HURDLE STEP	0	1	2	3
SHOULDER MOBILITY	0	1	2	3
ACTIVE STRAIGHT LEG RAISE	0	1	2	3
TRUNK STABILITY PUSH UP	0	1	2	3
ROTATIONAL STABILITY	0	1	2	3

0: You feel any pain at all

1: You can do the move, but not very well

2. You can do the move, but you need to compensate in some way.

3. You can perfectly master the move.

NUTRITION   GOAL

TOTAL CALORIES: _____   _____

GRAMS OF PROTEIN: _____   _____

HYDRATION: _____   _____

READING: _____

RESEARCH: _____

Date:
Focus: Endurance

SLEEP   Total Time   _____

                Quality   1   2   3   4   5

MOBILITY

ENDURANCE - 3x3   3 mile ruck   45 pounds

             Time: _____

                    100 Squats   with ruck

      Run   3 mile run

             Time: _____

                    100 Squats   without ruck

Cognition Prompt (KIMS Game): Commit this list of random items to memory.
1. Washing Machine 2. Sunglasses 3. Fence 4. Headphones 5. Bouquet 6. Shovel 7. Coat Hanger 8. Fork 9. Eyebrow 10. Shotgun

---

Socks: _____   Boots: _____

Hotspots: _____

NUTRITION   GOAL

             TOTAL CALORIES: _____ _____

          GRAMS OF PROTEIN: _____ _____

                  HYDRATION: _____ _____

READING: _____

RESEARCH: _____

WEEK 21 - DAY 3
Date:
Focus: Strength & Endurance

SLEEP   Total Time   _____

               Quality   1   2   3   4   5

MOBILITY

STRENGTH   80% 1RM   3 Sets   10-15 Reps

	Wt	/	Reps	Wt	/	Reps	Wt	/	Reps
Bench									
Row									
Shrug									

1-2 minutes rest between sets

ENDURANCE   45 min run   Zone 2

               Mileage: _____

               Avg HR: _____

NUTRITION   GOAL

        TOTAL CALORIES: _____ _____

    GRAMS OF PROTEIN: _____ _____

            HYDRATION: _____ _____

READING: _____

RESEARCH: _____

WEEK 21 – DAY 4
Date:
Focus: Endurance

SLEEP   Total Time   _____

            Quality   1   2   3   4   5

MOBILITY

ENDURANCE - 3x3   3 mile ruck   45 pounds

                    Time: _____

                          100 Squats   with ruck

            Run   3 mile run

                    Time: _____

                          100 Squats   without ruck

Cognition Prompt: Complete this creativity exercise.
Select two random objects or items. Combine them into a new product. Develop a vision or strategy to 'sell' this new item to others. How would you convince them of the importance of this innovative item? What things would you attempt to appeal to in order to get them bought in?

Socks: _____   Boots: _____
Hotspots: _____

NUTRITION   GOAL
            TOTAL CALORIES: _____ _____
            GRAMS OF PROTEIN: _____ _____
            HYDRATION: _____ _____

READING: _____

RESEARCH: _____

WEEK 21 - DAY 5
Date:
Focus: Strength

SLEEP   Total Time   _____

            Quality   1   2   3   4   5

MOBILITY

STRENGTH   80% 1RM   3 Sets   10-15 Reps

SQUAT Wt / Reps Wt / Reps Wt / Reps

DEADLIFT Wt / Reps Wt / Reps Wt / Reps

OHP Wt / Reps Wt / Reps Wt / Reps

1-2 minutes rest between sets

NUTRITION   GOAL

TOTAL CALORIES: _____ _____

GRAMS OF PROTEIN: _____ _____

HYDRATION: _____ _____

READING: _____

RESEARCH: _____

SLEEP   Total Time   _____
                     Quality   1   2   3   4   5

MOBILITY

SKILLS   From Menu

NUTRITION   GOAL
               TOTAL CALORIES: _____ _____
            GRAMS OF PROTEIN: _____ _____
                    HYDRATION: _____ _____

READING: _____

RESEARCH: _____

WEEK 21 – DAY 7
Date:
Focus: Rest

SLEEP   Total Time   _____

              Quality   1   2   3   4   5

MOBILITY

SUMMARY	SLEEP	CALORIES	PROTEIN	HYDRATION
Day 1				
Day 2				
Day 3				
Day 4				
Day 5				
Day 6				
Day 7				

NUTRITION   GOAL

TOTAL CALORIES: _____ _____

GRAMS OF PROTEIN: _____ _____

HYDRATION: _____ _____

NEXT WEEK TRAINING FOCUS: _____

_____

_____

MOBILITY WORKSHEET

WEEK 22 - SUMMARY

We are moving up to a 3x3 and we are adding weight to the ruck to bring it up to 50 pounds. You will feel the difference in distance and weight. Enjoy it. This pressure is your constant friend. Greet him like an old pal and welcome him to your existence. Embrace the suck.

DAY 1	MOBILITY 1	STRENGTH WORK
DAY 2	MOBILITY 2	ENDURANCE WORK
DAY 3	MOBILITY 1	STRENGTH & ENDURANCE
DAY 4	MOBILITY 2	ENDURANCE WORK
DAY 5	MOBILITY 1	STRENGTH & SPEED
DAY 6	MOBILITY 2	ENDURANCE WORK
DAY 7		REST

The content of your character is your choice. Day by day, what you choose, what you think, and what you do is who you become. – Heraclitus

WEEK 22 - DAY 1
Date:
Focus: Strength

SLEEP   Total Time   _____
              Quality   1   2   3   4   5

MOBILITY

STRENGTH   85% 1RM   4 Sets   8-10 Reps

	Wt	/	Reps	Wt	/	Reps	Wt	/	Reps	Wt	/	Reps
Bench												
Row												
Shrug												

2-4 minutes rest between sets

NUTRITION   GOAL
        TOTAL CALORIES: _____ _____
    GRAMS OF PROTEIN: _____ _____
          HYDRATION: _____ _____

READING: _____

RESEARCH: _____

Date:
Focus: Endurance

SLEEP   Total Time   _____
          Quality   1   2   3   4   5

MOBILITY

ENDURANCE - 3x3   3 mile ruck   50 pounds
                    Time: _____
                              100 Squats   with ruck
          Run   3 mile run
                    Time: _____
                              100 Squats   without ruck

Cognition Prompt: Complete this creativity exercise.

Develop a 6-word story. Once you've created the story, allow yourself to think about the details
of the story. Fill in the gaps. Repeat this as many times as necessary until you've completed
your training session for the day.

Socks: _____   Boots: _____
Hotspots: _____

NUTRITION   GOAL
          TOTAL CALORIES: _____ _____
          GRAMS OF PROTEIN: _____ _____
          HYDRATION: _____ _____

READING: _____

RESEARCH: _____

WEEK 22 - DAY 3
Date:
Focus: Strength and Endurance

SLEEP   Total Time   _____

             Quality   1   2   3   4   5

MOBILITY

STRENGTH   85% 1RM   4 Sets   8-10 Reps

	Wt	/	Reps	Wt	/	Reps	Wt	/	Reps	Wt	/	Reps
Squat												
Deadlift												
OHP												

2-4 minutes rest between sets

ENDURANCE   45 min run   Zone 2

            Mileage: _____

            Avg HR: _____

NUTRITION   GOAL

        TOTAL CALORIES: _____ _____

    GRAMS OF PROTEIN: _____ _____

           HYDRATION: _____ _____

READING: _____

RESEARCH: _____

WEEK 22 - DAY 4
Date:
Focus: Endurance

SLEEP   Total Time   _____

             Quality   1   2   3   4   5

MOBILITY

ENDURANCE - 3x3   3 mile ruck   50 pounds

                     Time: _____

                             100 Squats   with ruck

             Run   3 mile run

                     Time: _____

                             100 Squats   without ruck

Cognition Prompt: What information can you gather using your sense of smell? What do you smell and how does it change over time? Whenever these sensations retreat to the background, consciously become aware of the things that you smell.

Socks: _____   Boots: _____
Hotspots: _____

NUTRITION   GOAL
             TOTAL CALORIES: _____ _____
             GRAMS OF PROTEIN: _____ _____
             HYDRATION: _____ _____

READING: _____

RESEARCH: _____

Date:
Focus: Strength

SLEEP   Total Time   _____
             Quality   1   2   3   4   5

MOBILITY

STRENGTH   85% 1RM   4 Sets   8-10 Reps

Bench Wt / Reps   Wt / Reps   Wt / Reps   Wt / Reps
_____

Row   Wt / Reps   Wt / Reps   Wt / Reps   Wt / Reps
_____

Shrug Wt / Reps   Wt / Reps   Wt / Reps   Wt / Reps
_____

2-4 minutes rest between sets

NUTRITION   GOAL
            TOTAL CALORIES: _____   _____
         GRAMS OF PROTEIN: _____   _____
                HYDRATION: _____   _____

READING: _____

RESEARCH: _____

WEEK 22 - DAY 6
Date:
Focus: Endurance

SLEEP   Total Time   _____
             Quality   1   2   3   4   5

MOBILITY

ENDURANCE - 3x3   3 mile ruck   50 pounds
                    Time: _____
                           100 Squats   with ruck
             Run   3 mile run
                    Time: _____
                           100 Squats   without ruck

Cognition Prompt: Reflect on the past week.
What would you change?
Where did you cut corners?
What did you do well and need to continue doing?

Socks: _____   Boots: _____
Hotspots: _____

NUTRITION   GOAL
        TOTAL CALORIES: _____ _____
      GRAMS OF PROTEIN: _____ _____
             HYDRATION: _____ _____

READING: _____

RESEARCH: _____

WEEK 22 - DAY 7
Date:
Focus: Rest

SLEEP   Total Time   _____
              Quality   1   2   3   4   5

MOBILITY

SUMMARY	SLEEP	CALORIES	PROTEIN	HYDRATION
Day 1				
Day 2				
Day 3				
Day 4				
Day 5				
Day 6				
Day 7				

NUTRITION   GOAL
          TOTAL CALORIES: _____   _____
        GRAMS OF PROTEIN: _____   _____
               HYDRATION: _____   _____

NEXT WEEK TRAINING FOCUS: _____

_____
_____

WEEK 23 - SUMMARY

We bump up to a 3x4, the ruck weight stays the same and we do another skills session. Keep grinding. You can cuss the whole time but keep grinding.

DAY 1	MOBILITY 1	STRENGTH WORK
DAY 2	MOBILITY 2	ENDURANCE WORK
DAY 3	MOBILITY 1	STRENGTH & ENDURANCE
DAY 4	MOBILITY 2	ENDURANCE WORK
DAY 5	MOBILITY 1	STRENGTH WORK
DAY 6	MOBILITY 2	SKILLS WORK
DAY 7		REST

Stand in the gap. A Green Beret stands in the gap between freedom and oppression and says, "No matter what happens, nothing is getting by me." And the Brotherhood stands with him and says, "Nothing is getting by *us*."

WEEK 23 - DAY 1
Date:
Focus: Strength

<u>SLEEP</u>   Total Time   _____
            Quality   1   2   3   4   5

<u>MOBILITY</u>

<u>STRENGTH</u>   85% 1RM   4 Sets   8-10 Reps

Squat Wt / Reps Wt / Reps Wt / Reps Wt / Reps

Deadlift Wt / Reps Wt / Reps Wt / Reps Wt / Reps

OHP Wt / Reps Wt / Reps Wt / Reps Wt / Reps

2-4 minutes rest between sets

<u>NUTRITION</u>   GOAL
    TOTAL CALORIES: _____ _____
    GRAMS OF PROTEIN: _____ _____
    HYDRATION: _____ _____

READING: _____

RESEARCH: _____

WEEK 23 - DAY 2
Date:
Focus: Endurance

SLEEP   Total Time   _____

          Quality   1   2   3   4   5

MOBILITY

ENDURANCE - 3x4   3 mile ruck   50 pounds

                    Time: _____

                         100 Squats   with ruck

          Run   4 mile run

                    Time: _____

                         100 Squats   without ruck

Cognition Prompt (KIMS Game): Commit this list of military items to memory.

1. Compass 2. Notebook 3. Canteen 4. Ammunition 5. Woobie 6. C-Wire 7. First-Aid Kit 8. NVGs

Socks: _____   Boots: _____

Hotspots: _____

NUTRITION   GOAL

          TOTAL CALORIES: _____ _____

          GRAMS OF PROTEIN: _____ _____

          HYDRATION: _____ _____

READING: _____

RESEARCH: _____

WEEK 23 - DAY 3
Date:
Focus: Strength and Endurance

SLEEP   Total Time   _____

                 Quality   1   2   3   4   5

MOBILITY

STRENGTH   85% 1RM   4 Sets   8-10 Reps

	Wt	/	Reps	Wt	/	Reps	Wt	/	Reps	Wt	/	Reps
Bench												
Row												
Shrug												

2-4 minutes rest between sets

ENDURANCE   45 min run   Zone 2

                 Mileage: _____

                 Avg HR: _____

NUTRITION   GOAL

         TOTAL CALORIES: _____ _____

    GRAMS OF PROTEIN: _____ _____

             HYDRATION: _____ _____

READING: _____

RESEARCH: _____

SLEEP   Total Time   _____

             Quality   1   2   3   4   5

MOBILITY

ENDURANCE - 3x4   3 mile ruck   50 pounds

             Time: _____

             100 Squats   with ruck

        Run   4 mile run

             Time: _____

             100 Squats   without ruck

Cognition Prompt: Complete this creativity exercise.

Attempt to think in a way that eliminates the words: "I", "Me", "My", and "Mine". Broaden the way in which you interact with your mind and the dialogue it generates.

Socks: _____   Boots: _____

Hotspots: _____

NUTRITION   GOAL

        TOTAL CALORIES: _____   _____

    GRAMS OF PROTEIN: _____   _____

            HYDRATION: _____   _____

READING: _____

RESEARCH: _____

Date:
Focus: Strength

SLEEP   Total Time   _____
              Quality   1   2   3   4   5

MOBILITY

STRENGTH   85% 1RM   4 Sets   8-10 Reps

	Wt / Reps	Wt / Reps	Wt / Reps	Wt / Reps
Squat				
Deadlift				
OHP				

2-4 minutes rest between sets

NUTRITION   GOAL
        TOTAL CALORIES: _____ _____
    GRAMS OF PROTEIN: _____ _____
           HYDRATION: _____ _____

READING: _____

RESEARCH: _____

WEEK 23 - DAY 6
Date:
Focus: Skills

SLEEP   Total Time   _____

             Quality   1   2   3   4   5

MOBILITY

SKILLS   From Menu

NUTRITION   GOAL

        TOTAL CALORIES: _____ _____

    GRAMS OF PROTEIN: _____ _____

           HYDRATION: _____ _____

READING: _____

RESEARCH: _____

WEEK 23 - DAY 7
Date:
Focus: Rest

SLEEP   Total Time   _____
             Quality   1   2   3   4   5

MOBILITY

SUMMARY	SLEEP	CALORIES	PROTEIN	HYDRATION
Day 1				
Day 2				
Day 3				
Day 4				
Day 5				
Day 6				
Day 7				

NUTRITION   GOAL
            TOTAL CALORIES: _____ _____
         GRAMS OF PROTEIN: _____ _____
                HYDRATION: _____ _____

NEXT WEEK TRAINING FOCUS: _____

_____
_____

WEEK 24 - SUMMARY

We are violating the "do not increase weight, distance or pace by more than 10% week to week" axiom. Enjoy it.

DAY 1	MOBILITY 1	STRENGTH WORK
DAY 2	MOBILITY 2	ENDURANCE WORK
DAY 3	MOBILITY 1	STRENGTH & RECOVERY
DAY 4	MOBILITY 2	ENDURANCE WORK
DAY 5	MOBILITY 1	STRENGTH WORK
DAY 6	MOBILITY 2	ENDURANCE WORK
DAY 7		REST

The true man is revealed in difficult times. - Epictetus

Date:

Focus: Strength

SLEEP   Total Time   _____

Quality   1   2   3   4   5

MOBILITY

STRENGTH   85% 1RM   4 Sets   8-10 Reps

Bench   Wt   /   Reps   Wt   /   Reps   Wt   /   Reps   Wt   /   Reps
_____

Row   Wt   /   Reps   Wt   /   Reps   Wt   /   Reps   Wt   /   Reps
_____

Shrug   Wt   /   Reps   Wt   /   Reps   Wt   /   Reps   Wt   /   Reps
_____

2-4 minutes rest between sets

NUTRITION   GOAL

TOTAL CALORIES: _____   _____

GRAMS OF PROTEIN: _____   _____

HYDRATION: _____   _____

READING: _____

RESEARCH: _____

WEEK 24 - DAY 2
Date:
Focus: Endurance

SLEEP   Total Time   _____

              Quality   1   2   3   4   5

MOBILITY

ENDURANCE - 3x4   3 mile ruck   50 pounds

              Time: _____

                             100 Squats   with ruck

              Run   4 mile run

              Time: _____

                             100 Squats   without ruck

Cognition Prompt: Allow your mind to get lost on something in your surroundings. Find something that interests you, it can be anything at all. Generate questions about that thing, study it and pick out details about it. See how long your mind will linger on that feature of your environment until it is ready to find something new. Repeat this with different objects around you until your PT is complete

Socks: _____   Boots: _____

Hotspots: _____

NUTRITION   GOAL

              TOTAL CALORIES: _____ _____

              GRAMS OF PROTEIN: _____ _____

              HYDRATION: _____ _____

READING: _____

RESEARCH: _____

WEEK 24 - DAY 3
Date:
Focus: Strength and Recovery

SLEEP   Total Time   _____

              Quality   1   2   3   4   5

MOBILITY

STRENGTH   85% 1RM   4 Sets   8-10 Reps

Squat	Wt / Reps	Wt / Reps	Wt / Reps	Wt / Reps
Deadlift	Wt / Reps	Wt / Reps	Wt / Reps	Wt / Reps
OHP	Wt / Reps	Wt / Reps	Wt / Reps	Wt / Reps

2-4 minutes rest between sets

ENDURANCE   45 min run   Zone 1

              Mileage: _____   Recovery

              Avg HR: _____

NUTRITION   GOAL

        TOTAL CALORIES: _____ _____

     GRAMS OF PROTEIN: _____ _____

             HYDRATION: _____ _____

READING: _____

RESEARCH: _____

WEEK 24 - DAY 4
Date:
Focus: Endurance

SLEEP   Total Time   _____

              Quality   1   2   3   4   5

MOBILITY

ENDURANCE - 3x4   3 mile ruck   50 pounds

                    Time: _____

                             100 Squats   with ruck

              Run   4 mile run

                    Time: _____

                             100 Squats   without ruck

Cognition Prompt: If you had a gun to your head and had to identify one moment in your life
where you would do something differently, what would that one moment be?
Why would you seek to change it, and what would you do?

Socks: _____   Boots: _____

Hotspots: _____

NUTRITION   GOAL

              TOTAL CALORIES: _____   _____

           GRAMS OF PROTEIN: _____   _____

                  HYDRATION: _____   _____

READING: _____

RESEARCH: _____

WEEK 24 - DAY 5
Date:
Focus: Strength

SLEEP   Total Time   _____
              Quality   1   2   3   4   5

MOBILITY

STRENGTH   85% 1RM   4 Sets   8-10 Reps

Bench   Wt   /   Reps   Wt   /   Reps   Wt   /   Reps   Wt   /   Reps
_____

Row   Wt   /   Reps   Wt   /   Reps   Wt   /   Reps   Wt   /   Reps
_____

Shrug   Wt   /   Reps   Wt   /   Reps   Wt   /   Reps   Wt   /   Reps
_____

2-4 minutes rest between sets

NUTRITION   GOAL
          TOTAL CALORIES: _____   _____
        GRAMS OF PROTEIN: _____   _____
              HYDRATION: _____   _____

READING: _____

RESEARCH: _____

SLEEP

Total Time _____

Quality   1   2   3   4   5

MOBILITY

ENDURANCE - 3x4

                   3 mile ruck   50 pounds

          Time: _____

                   100 Squats   with ruck

      Run   4 mile run

          Time: _____

                   100 Squats   without ruck

Cognition Prompt: Remember each of the primary missions of Special Forces:

1. Unconventional Warfare 2. Foreign Internal Defense 3. Special Reconnaissance 4. Direct Action 5. Combat Terrorism

Socks: _____   Boots: _____

Hotspots: _____

NUTRITION

                                                    GOAL

TOTAL CALORIES: _____ _____

GRAMS OF PROTEIN: _____ _____

HYDRATION: _____ _____

READING: _____

RESEARCH: _____

WEEK 24 – DAY 7
Date:
Focus: Rest

SLEEP Total Time   _____
          Quality   1   2   3   4   5

MOBILITY

SUMMARY	SLEEP	CALORIES	PROTEIN	HYDRATION
Day 1				
Day 2				
Day 3				
Day 4				
Day 5				
Day 6				
Day 7				

NUTRITION   GOAL

TOTAL CALORIES: _____ _____

GRAMS OF PROTEIN: _____ _____

HYDRATION: _____ _____

NEXT WEEK TRAINING FOCUS: _____

_____

_____

WEEK 25 - SUMMARY

We will re-establish our 1 RM so that we can close out the program on a clean sheet. We will also take a 12 mile ruck assessment and we bump up to a 4x4.

DAY 1	MOBILITY 1	ETABLISH 1RM
DAY 2	MOBILITY 2	ENDURANCE WORK
DAY 3	MOBILITY 1	STRENGTH & RECOVERY
DAY 4	MOBILITY 2	ENDURANCE WORK
DAY 5	MOBILITY 1	STRENGTH WORK
DAY 6	MOBILITY 2	12 MILE RUCK
DAY 7		REST

Do you feel that weight? Do you feel the burden of your task? The pressure? The stress? That's a gift. You are meant to bear that burden. It is your duty. Great men are required to build great societies. Earn your place and bear that burden with pride. Be thankful for the gift. You are the foundation.
Lay yourself down and bear that responsibility.
This is where you are meant to be.

WEEK 25 - DAY 1
Date:
Focus: Strength & Assessment

SLEEP   Total Time   _____

              Quality   1   2   3   4   5

MOBILITY

STRENGTH

                  SQUAT   _____

               DEADLIFT   _____

                 BENCH   _____

                    ROW   _____

                 SHRUG   _____

                   OHP   _____

NUTRITION   GOAL

        TOTAL CALORIES: _____ _____

     GRAMS OF PROTEIN: _____ _____

            HYDRATION: _____ _____

READING: _____

RESEARCH: _____

WEEK 25 - DAY 2
Date:
Focus: Endurance

SLEEP   Total Time   _____

Quality   1   2   3   4   5

MOBILITY

ENDURANCE - 4x4   4 mile ruck   50 pounds

Time: _____

100 Squats   with ruck

Run   4 mile run

Time: _____

100 Squats   without ruck

Cognition Prompt: Remember each phase of Unconventional Warfare & a corresponding description:

1. Preparation 2. Initial Contact 3. Infiltration 4. Organization 5. Build Up 6. Employment 7. Transition

Socks: _____   Boots: _____

Hotspots: _____

NUTRITION   GOAL

TOTAL CALORIES: _____ _____

GRAMS OF PROTEIN: _____ _____

HYDRATION: _____ _____

READING: _____

RESEARCH: _____

WEEK 25 - DAY 3
Date:
Focus: Strength and Recovery

SLEEP   Total Time   _____
             Quality   1   2   3   4   5

MOBILITY

STRENGTH   80% 1RM   3 Sets   10-15 Reps

SQUAT Wt / Reps Wt / Reps Wt / Reps

DEADLIFT Wt / Reps Wt / Reps Wt / Reps

OHP Wt / Reps Wt / Reps Wt / Reps

1-2 minutes rest between sets

ENDURANCE   35 min run   Zone 1
                Mileage: _____   Recovery
                Avg HR: _____

NUTRITION   GOAL
            TOTAL CALORIES: _____   _____
          GRAMS OF PROTEIN: _____   _____
                HYDRATION: _____   _____

READING: _____

RESEARCH: _____

SLEEP   Total Time   _____

Quality   1   2   3   4   5

MOBILITY

ENDURANCE - 4x4   4 mile ruck   50 pounds

Time: _____

100 Squats   with ruck

Run   4 mile run

Time: _____

100 Squats   without ruck

Cognition Prompt: Study any other people who you encounter today during your workout. As you pass them or see them, make a point to focus on their facial features (clothing, height, eight, etc.). What are the things that stand out to you? What inferences might you make about this person? Would you be able to pick them out in a crowd if you saw them again?

Socks: _____   Boots: _____

Hotspots: _____

NUTRITION   GOAL

TOTAL CALORIES: _____ _____

GRAMS OF PROTEIN: _____ _____

HYDRATION: _____ _____

READING: _____

RESEARCH: _____

Date:
Focus: Strength

SLEEP Total Time _____
Quality   1   2   3   4   5

MOBILITY

STRENGTH   80% 1RM   3 Sets   10-15 Reps

Bench Wt / Reps Wt / Reps Wt / Reps
_____

Row Wt / Reps Wt / Reps Wt / Reps
_____

Shrug Wt / Reps Wt / Reps Wt / Reps
_____

1-2 minutes rest between sets

NUTRITION   GOAL
          TOTAL CALORIES: _____ _____
        GRAMS OF PROTEIN: _____ _____
              HYDRATION: _____ _____

READING: _____

RESEARCH: _____

WEEK 25 - DAY 6
Date:
Focus: 12 Mile Ruck Assessment

SLEEP   Total Time   _____

              Quality   1   2   3   4   5

MOBILITY

RUCK   12 Miles

              TIME _____

     AVERAGE HR: _____

Cognition Prompt: Complete this creativity exercise.

Pick someone in your life who you deeply care about. Attempt to put yourself in his or her shoes. How do they feel about your preparation for SFAS? What does it look like from their perspective? Do they understand why you are striving towards this goal? How do they view your actions and choices?

BOOTS   _____

SOCKS   _____

HOT SPOTS _____

PAIN POINTS _____

NUTRITION   GOAL

        TOTAL CALORIES: _____ ____

       GRAMS OF PROTEIN: _____ ____

           HYDRATION: _____ ____

READING: _____

RESEARCH: _____

WEEK 25 - DAY 7
Date:
Focus: Rest

SLEEP   Total Time   _____

Quality   1   2   3   4   5

MOBILITY

SUMMARY	SLEEP	CALORIES	PROTEIN	HYDRATION
Day 1				
Day 2				
Day 3				
Day 4				
Day 5				
Day 6				
Day 7				

NUTRITION   GOAL

TOTAL CALORIES: _____ _____

GRAMS OF PROTEIN: _____ _____

HYDRATION: _____ _____

NEXT WEEK TRAINING FOCUS: _____

_____

_____

WEEK 26 - SUMMARY

This is a deload week. You put in 20 miles under a ruck last week, so we will take a short break with only 8 this week. It is all uphill from here.

DAY 1	MOBILITY 1	STRENGTH WORK
DAY 2	MOBILITY 2	ENDURANCE WORK
DAY 3	MOBILITY 1	STRENGTH & RECOVERY
DAY 4	MOBILITY 2	ENDURANCE WORK
DAY 5	MOBILITY 1	STRENGTH & SPEED
DAY 6	MOBILITY 2	SKILLS WORK
DAY 7		REST

The harder you work, the luckier you get.

WEEK 26 - DAY 1
Date:
Focus: Strength

SLEEP   Total Time   _____
              Quality   1   2   3   4   5

MOBILITY

STRENGTH   80% 1RM   3 Sets   10-15 Reps

SQUAT   Wt   /   Reps   Wt   /   Reps   Wt   /   Reps

DEADLIFT   Wt   /   Reps   Wt   /   Reps   Wt   /   Reps

OHP   Wt   /   Reps   Wt   /   Reps   Wt   /   Reps

1-2 minutes rest between sets

NUTRITION   GOAL
                 TOTAL CALORIES: _____ _____
          GRAMS OF PROTEIN: _____ _____
                     HYDRATION: _____ _____

READING: _____

RESEARCH: _____

WEEK 26 - DAY 2
Date:
Focus: Endurance

SLEEP   Total Time   _____
              Quality   1   2   3   4   5

MOBILITY

ENDURANCE - 4x4   4 mile ruck   50 pounds
                Time: _____
                           100 Squats   with ruck
              Run   4 mile run
                Time: _____
                           100 Squats   without ruck

Cognition Prompt: Train the shift between situational awareness and self awareness. Imagine three general levels for your mind to attune to: your breath, your body, your external environment. Intentionally shift your attention between each of these 3 specific stages of knowing. Focus on the breath. Shift to focusing on your body with a complete body scan. Shift to the world around you. Repeat this process, aiming to make each shift as efficient as possible.

Socks: _____   Boots: _____
Hotspots: _____

NUTRITION   GOAL
            TOTAL CALORIES: _____ _____
          GRAMS OF PROTEIN: _____ _____
                 HYDRATION: _____ _____

READING: _____

RESEARCH: _____

WEEK 26 - DAY 3
Date:
Focus: Strength and Endurance

SLEEP   Total Time   _____

            Quality   1   2   3   4   5

MOBILITY

STRENGTH   80% 1RM   3 Sets   10-15 Reps

Bench Wt / Reps Wt / Reps Wt / Reps

Row Wt / Reps Wt / Reps Wt / Reps

Shrug Wt / Reps Wt / Reps Wt / Reps

1-2 minutes rest between sets

ENDURANCE   35 min run   Zone 1

           Mileage: _____   Recovery

           Avg HR: _____

NUTRITION   GOAL

          TOTAL CALORIES: _____ _____

      GRAMS OF PROTEIN: _____ _____

              HYDRATION: _____ _____

READING: _____

RESEARCH: _____

WEEK 26 - DAY 4
Date:
Focus: Endurance

SLEEP   Total Time   _____

            Quality   1   2   3   4   5

MOBILITY

ENDURANCE - 4x4   4 mile ruck   50 pounds

               Time: _____

                    100 Squats   with ruck

        Run   4 mile run

               Time: _____

                    100 Squats   without ruck

Cognition Prompt: Observe your surroundings as if you were a cartographer. Observe the changes in elevations and the landmarks in your environment. What would these look like if you were reading a map? Visualize it clearly in your mind's eye.

Socks: _____   Boots: _____

Hotspots: _____

NUTRITION   GOAL

           TOTAL CALORIES: _____ _____

      GRAMS OF PROTEIN: _____ _____

               HYDRATION: _____ _____

READING: _____

RESEARCH: _____

WEEK 26 - DAY 5
Date:
Focus: Strength

SLEEP   Total Time   _____

           Quality   1   2   3   4   5

MOBILITY

STRENGTH   80% 1RM   3 Sets   10-15 Reps

SQUAT Wt / Reps Wt / Reps Wt / Reps

DEADLIFT Wt / Reps Wt / Reps Wt / Reps

OHP Wt / Reps Wt / Reps Wt / Reps

1-2 minutes rest between sets

SPEED   Run   8 x 400 - Z4

                              1:2 work:rest

NUTRITION   GOAL

        TOTAL CALORIES: _____ _____

    GRAMS OF PROTEIN: _____ _____

           HYDRATION: _____ _____

READING: _____

RESEARCH: _____

SLEEP Total Time   _____
           Quality   1   2   3   4   5

MOBILITY

SKILLS   From Menu

NUTRITION   GOAL
         TOTAL CALORIES: _____ _____
       GRAMS OF PROTEIN: _____ _____
             HYDRATION: _____ _____

READING: _____

RESEARCH: _____

WEEK 26 - DAY 7
Date:
Focus: Rest

SLEEP   Total Time   _____

                   Quality   1   2   3   4   5

MOBILITY

SUMMARY	SLEEP	CALORIES	PROTEIN	HYDRATION
Day 1				
Day 2				
Day 3				
Day 4				
Day 5				
Day 6				
Day 7				

NUTRITION   GOAL

           TOTAL CALORIES: _____ _____

     GRAMS OF PROTEIN: _____ _____

                HYDRATION: _____ _____

NEXT WEEK TRAINING FOCUS: _____

WEEK 27 - SUMMARY

Fast week. Simple schedule. We bump up to a 4x5. Earn it.

DAY 1	MOBILITY 1	STRENGTH WORK
DAY 2	MOBILITY 2	ENDURANCE WORK
DAY 3	MOBILITY 1	STRENGTH WORK
DAY 4	MOBILITY 2	ENDURANCE WORK
DAY 5	MOBILITY 1	STRENGTH WORK
DAY 6	MOBILITY 2	ENDURANCE WORK
DAY 7		REST

One more. That's the only way. One more rep. One more set. One more lap. One more day. Hold on for one more day. One more.

WEEK 27 - DAY 1
Date:
Focus: Strength

SLEEP   Total Time   _____

            Quality   1   2   3   4   5

MOBILITY

STRENGTH   80% 1RM   3 Sets   10-15 Reps

Bench Wt / Reps Wt / Reps Wt / Reps

Row Wt / Reps Wt / Reps Wt / Reps

Shrug Wt / Reps Wt / Reps Wt / Reps

1-2 minutes rest between sets

NUTRITION   GOAL

TOTAL CALORIES: _____ ____

GRAMS OF PROTEIN: _____ ____

HYDRATION: _____ ____

READING: _____

RESEARCH: _____

SLEEP   Total Time   _____
              Quality   1   2   3   4   5

MOBILITY

ENDURANCE - 4x5   4 mile ruck   50 pounds
                    Time: _____
                             100 Squats   with ruck
              Run   5 mile run
                    Time: _____
                             100 Squats   without ruck

Cognition Prompt: If (when) you achieve your goal of successful selection to Special forces, how would you change as a result?
What would you DO differently from that point on? How would you act or feel differently?

Socks: _____   Boots: _____
Hotspots: _____

NUTRITION   GOAL
              TOTAL CALORIES: _____ _____
              GRAMS OF PROTEIN: _____ _____
              HYDRATION: _____ _____

READING: _____

RESEARCH: _____

SLEEP   Total Time   _____

Quality   1   2   3   4   5

MOBILITY

STRENGTH   80% 1RM   3 Sets   10-15 Reps

SQUAT Wt / Reps Wt / Reps Wt / Reps
_____

DEADLIFT Wt / Reps Wt / Reps Wt / Reps
_____

OHP Wt / Reps Wt / Reps Wt / Reps
_____

1-2 minutes rest between sets

ENDURANCE   35 min run   Zone 1

Mileage: _____   Recovery

Avg HR: _____

NUTRITION   GOAL

TOTAL CALORIES: _____ _____

GRAMS OF PROTEIN: _____ _____

HYDRATION: _____ _____

READING: _____

RESEARCH: _____

WEEK 27 - DAY 4
Date:
Focus: Endurance

SLEEP   Total Time   _____
             Quality   1   2   3   4   5

MOBILITY

ENDURANCE - 4x5   4 mile ruck   50 pounds
                Time: _____
                            100 Squats   with ruck
             Run   5 mile run
                Time: _____
                            100 Squats   without ruck

Cognition Prompt: Remember each step of the Troop Leading Procedures in order:

1. Receive the Mission 2. Issue Warning Order 3. Make a Tentative Plan 4. Initiate Movement 5. Conduct Reconnaissance 6. Complete the Plan 7. Issue Operation Order 8. Supervise and Refine

Socks: _____   Boots: _____
Hotspots: _____

NUTRITION   GOAL
          TOTAL CALORIES: _____ _____
        GRAMS OF PROTEIN: _____ _____
              HYDRATION: _____ _____

READING: _____

RESEARCH: _____

WEEK 27 - DAY 5
Date:
Focus: Strength

<u>SLEEP</u>   Total Time   _____

Quality   1   2   3   4   5

<u>MOBILITY</u>

<u>STRENGTH</u>   80% 1RM   3 Sets   10-15 Reps

Bench Wt / Reps Wt / Reps Wt / Reps
_____

Row Wt / Reps Wt / Reps Wt / Reps
_____

Shrug Wt / Reps Wt / Reps Wt / Reps
_____

1-2 minutes rest between sets

<u>NUTRITION</u>   GOAL

TOTAL CALORIES: _____ _____

GRAMS OF PROTEIN: _____ _____

HYDRATION: _____ _____

READING: _____

RESEARCH: _____

WEEK 27 - DAY 6
Date:
Focus: Endurance

SLEEP   Total Time   _____
              Quality   1   2   3   4   5

MOBILITY

ENDURANCE - 4x5   4 mile ruck   50 pounds
                  Time: _____
                        100 Squats   with ruck
         Run   5 mile run
                  Time: _____
                        100 Squats   without ruck

Cognition Prompt: Complete this creativity exercise.

Come with a new thought, idea, observation, etc. every minute on the minute. There are no rules or parameters around what you come up with. The goal is just to generate something new each minute of your training session.

Socks: _____   Boots: _____
Hotspots: _____

NUTRITION   GOAL
            TOTAL CALORIES: _____ _____
          GRAMS OF PROTEIN: _____ _____
                 HYDRATION: _____ _____

READING: _____

RESEARCH: _____

WEEK 27 - DAY 7
Date:
Focus: Rest

SLEEP   Total Time   _____
                Quality   1   2   3   4   5

MOBILITY

SUMMARY	SLEEP	CALORIES	PROTEIN	HYDRATION
Day 1				
Day 2				
Day 3				
Day 4				
Day 5				
Day 6				
Day 7				

NUTRITION   GOAL
            TOTAL CALORIES: _____ _____
          GRAMS OF PROTEIN: _____ _____
                 HYDRATION: _____ _____

NEXT WEEK TRAINING FOCUS: _____

_____
_____

WEEK 28 - SUMMARY

This is the final stretch. We max out the 5x5 with 55 pounds for the remainder of the program.

DAY 1	MOBILITY 1	STRENGTH WORK
DAY 2	MOBILITY 2	ENDURANCE WORK
DAY 3	MOBILITY 1	STRENGTH & RECOVERY
DAY 4	MOBILITY 2	ENDURANCE WORK
DAY 5	MOBILITY 1	STRENGTH & SPEED
DAY 6	MOBILITY 2	SKILLS WORK
DAY 7		REST

The problem with being is elite, is that once you've tasted it,
nothing else will satisfy you.

WEEK 28 - DAY 1
Date:
Focus: Strength

SLEEP   Total Time   _____

               Quality   1   2   3   4   5

MOBILITY

STRENGTH   80% 1RM   3 Sets   10-15 Reps

SQUAT Wt / Reps Wt / Reps Wt / Reps

DEADLIFT Wt / Reps Wt / Reps Wt / Reps

OHP Wt / Reps Wt / Reps Wt / Reps

1-2 minutes rest between sets

NUTRITION   GOAL

        TOTAL CALORIES: _____ _____

     GRAMS OF PROTEIN: _____ _____

            HYDRATION: _____ _____

READING: _____

RESEARCH: _____

WEEK 28 - DAY 2
Date:
Focus: Endurance

SLEEP   Total Time _____

            Quality   1   2   3   4   5

MOBILITY

ENDURANCE - 5x5   5 mile ruck   55 pounds

            Time: _____

                    100 Squats   with ruck

        Run   5 mile run

            Time: _____

                    100 Squats   without ruck

Cognition Prompt: Observe your surroundings as if you were prepping an ambush or raid. What are the features of the environment you could use to your advantage? What are the potential pitfalls of using this space? Do this exercise every ~400 meters as the terrain changes.

Socks: _____   Boots: _____

Hotspots: _____

NUTRITION   GOAL

        TOTAL CALORIES: _____ _____

      GRAMS OF PROTEIN: _____ _____

            HYDRATION: _____ _____

READING: _____

RESEARCH: _____

WEEK 28 - DAY 3
Date:
Focus: Strength and Endurance

SLEEP Total Time _____
           Quality   1   2   3   4   5

MOBILITY

STRENGTH   80% 1RM   3 Sets   10-15 Reps

Bench Wt / Reps Wt / Reps Wt / Reps
_____

Row Wt / Reps Wt / Reps Wt / Reps
_____

Shrug Wt / Reps Wt / Reps Wt / Reps
_____

1-2 minutes rest between sets

ENDURANCE   35 min run   Zone 1
                Mileage: _____   Recovery
                Avg HR: _____

NUTRITION   GOAL
        TOTAL CALORIES: _____ _____
      GRAMS OF PROTEIN: _____ _____
            HYDRATION: _____ _____

READING: _____

RESEARCH: _____

WEEK 28 - DAY 4
Date:
Focus: Endurance

SLEEP   Total Time   _____

           Quality   1   2   3   4   5

MOBILITY

ENDURANCE - 5x5   5 mile ruck   55 pounds

             Time: _____

                  100 Squats   with ruck

        Run   5 mile run

             Time: _____

                  100 Squats   without ruck

Cognition Prompt: Set your attention on the external environment around you. Each time your attention gets distracted or pulled away by something internal (i.e. a thought, sensation, memory, emotion, etc.), take note of it and re-direct to something nearby. As this continues to happen, try and place a simple label on that experience that is pulling you out of the present moment.

Socks: _____   Boots: _____

Hotspots: _____

NUTRITION   GOAL

        TOTAL CALORIES: _____ _____

    GRAMS OF PROTEIN: _____ _____

           HYDRATION: _____ _____

READING: _____

RESEARCH: _____

WEEK 28 - DAY 5
Date:
Focus: Strength

SLEEP   Total Time   _____

Quality   1   2   3   4   5

MOBILITY

STRENGTH   80% 1RM   3 Sets   10-15 Reps

SQUAT   Wt   /   Reps   Wt   /   Reps   Wt   /   Reps

DEADLIFT   Wt   /   Reps   Wt   /   Reps   Wt   /   Reps

OHP   Wt   /   Reps   Wt   /   Reps   Wt   /   Reps

1-2 minutes rest between sets

SPEED   Run   8 x 400 - Z4

1:2 work:rest

NUTRITION   GOAL

TOTAL CALORIES: _____   ____

GRAMS OF PROTEIN: _____   ____

HYDRATION: _____   ____

READING: _____

RESEARCH: _____

Date:

Focus: Skills

SLEEP   Total Time   _____

                Quality   1   2   3   4   5

MOBILITY

SKILLS   From Menu

NUTRITION   GOAL

          TOTAL CALORIES: _____ _____

     GRAMS OF PROTEIN: _____ _____

                HYDRATION: _____ _____

READING: _____

RESEARCH: _____

WEEK 28 – DAY 7
Date:
Focus: Rest

SLEEP   Total Time   _____

Quality   1   2   3   4   5

MOBILITY

SUMMARY	SLEEP	CALORIES	PROTEIN	HYDRATION
Day 1				
Day 2				
Day 3				
Day 4				
Day 5				
Day 6				
Day 7				

NUTRITION   GOAL

TOTAL CALORIES: _____ _____

GRAMS OF PROTEIN: _____ _____

HYDRATION: _____ _____

NEXT WEEK TRAINING FOCUS: _____

_____

WEEK 29 - SUMMARY

We will do our final PFA and FMS. You should be maxing or close to maxing the PFT and you should have no pain and full function in the FMS. You are strong and we will test that strength with a bump to 90% 1RM.

DAY 1	MOBILITY 1	ASSESSMENT
DAY 2	MOBILITY 2	ENDURANCE WORK
DAY 3	MOBILITY 1	STRENGTH & RECOVERY
DAY 4	MOBILITY 2	ENDURANCE WORK
DAY 5	MOBILITY 1	STRENGTH WORK
DAY 6	MOBILITY 2	SKILLS WORK
DAY 7		REST

There is no substitute for preparation.

WEEK 29 - DAY 1

Date:

Focus: Assessment

SLEEP   Total Time   _____

Quality   1   2   3   4   5

PFA   **HRPU**
     PLANK
     PULL-UPS
     2 MILE RUN

DEEP SQUAT	0	1	2	3
INLINE LUNGE	0	1	2	3
HURDLE STEP	0	1	2	3
SHOULDER MOBILITY	0	1	2	3
ACTIVE STRAIGHT LEG RAISE	0	1	2	3
TRUNK STABILITY PUSH UP	0	1	2	3
ROTATIONAL STABILITY	0	1	2	3

0: You feel any pain at all

1: You can do the move, but not very well

2. You can do the move, but you need to compensate in some way.

3. You can perfectly master the move.

NUTRITION   GOAL

TOTAL CALORIES: _____ _____

GRAMS OF PROTEIN: _____ _____

HYDRATION: _____ _____

READING: _____

RESEARCH: _____

Date:
Focus: Endurance

SLEEP   Total Time   _____

Quality   1   2   3   4   5

MOBILITY

ENDURANCE - 5x5   5 mile ruck   55 pounds

Time: _____

100 Squats   with ruck

Run   5 mile run

Time: _____

100 Squats   without ruck

Cognition Prompt: What are the primary forms of vegetation in this area? Can you spot different types of trees? What are the specific features of each type of vegetation that stand out to you? As you observe the plant life in your surroundings, what other features of your environment become more noticeable to you? How could you leverage this during different military tasks?

Socks: _____   Boots: _____

Hotspots: _____

NUTRITION   GOAL

TOTAL CALORIES: _____ _____

GRAMS OF PROTEIN: _____ _____

HYDRATION: _____ _____

READING: _____

RESEARCH: _____

Date:
Focus: Strength & Recovery

SLEEP   Total Time   _____
              Quality   1   2   3   4   5

MOBILITY

STRENGTH   90% 1RM   4 Sets   8-10 Reps

Squat   Wt / Reps   Wt / Reps   Wt / Reps   Wt / Reps

Deadlift Wt / Reps   Wt / Reps   Wt / Reps   Wt / Reps

OHP   Wt / Reps   Wt / Reps   Wt / Reps   Wt / Reps

2-4 minutes rest between sets

ENDURANCE   35 min run   Zone 1
              Mileage: _____   Recovery
              Avg HR: _____

NUTRITION   GOAL
        TOTAL CALORIES: _____ _____
     GRAMS OF PROTEIN: _____ _____
            HYDRATION: _____ _____

READING: _____

RESEARCH: _____

WEEK 29 - DAY 4
Date:
Focus: Endurance

SLEEP   Total Time   _____

                Quality   1   2   3   4   5

MOBILITY

ENDURANCE - 5x5   5 mile ruck   55 pounds

                    Time: _____

                             100 Squats   with ruck

            Run   5 mile run

                    Time: _____

                             100 Squats   without ruck

Cognition Prompt: Seeing what is missing can sometimes be as important as seeing what is there. As you navigate your surroundings, reflect on what is not present to your eye that you find surprising or interesting. As you identify potential things that are missing, question why that may be the case

Socks: _____   Boots: _____

Hotspots: _____

NUTRITION   GOAL

            TOTAL CALORIES: _____ _____

            GRAMS OF PROTEIN: _____ _____

            HYDRATION: _____ _____

READING: _____

RESEARCH: _____

WEEK 29 - DAY 5
Date:
Focus: Strength

SLEEP   Total Time   _____
Quality   1   2   3   4   5

MOBILITY

STRENGTH   90% 1RM   4 Sets   8-10 Reps

Bench   Wt   /   Reps   Wt   /   Reps   Wt   /   Reps   Wt   /   Reps
_____

Row   Wt   /   Reps   Wt   /   Reps   Wt   /   Reps   Wt   /   Reps
_____

Shrug   Wt   /   Reps   Wt   /   Reps   Wt   Reps   Wt   /   Reps
_____

2-4 minutes rest between sets

NUTRITION   GOAL
TOTAL CALORIES: _____   _____
GRAMS OF PROTEIN: _____   _____
HYDRATION: _____   _____

READING: _____

RESEARCH: _____

WEEK 29 - DAY 6
Date:
Focus: Skills

SLEEP   Total Time   _____
            Quality   1   2   3   4   5

MOBILITY

SKILLS   From Menu

NUTRITION   GOAL
        TOTAL CALORIES: _____ _____
    GRAMS OF PROTEIN: _____ _____
           HYDRATION: _____ _____

READING: _____

RESEARCH: _____

WEEK 29 - DAY 7
Date:
Focus: Rest

SLEEP   Total Time   _____

             Quality   1   2   3   4   5

MOBILITY

SUMMARY	SLEEP	CALORIES	PROTEIN	HYDRATION
Day 1				
Day 2				
Day 3				
Day 4				
Day 5				
Day 6				
Day 7				

NUTRITION   GOAL

        TOTAL CALORIES: _____ _____

    GRAMS OF PROTEIN: _____ _____

            HYDRATION: _____ _____

NEXT WEEK TRAINING FOCUS: _____

_____

_____

WEEK 30 - SUMMARY

3 rucks, 15 miles, 3 runs, 15 miles, and a recovery run. 3 strength sessions at 90% 1RM. The perfect week. Own it.

DAY 1	MOBILITY 1	STRENGTH WORK
DAY 2	MOBILITY 2	ENDURANCE WORK
DAY 3	MOBILITY 1	STRENGTH & RECOVERY
DAY 4	MOBILITY 2	ENDURANCE WORK
DAY 5	MOBILITY 1	STRENGTH WORK
DAY 6	MOBILITY 2	ENDURANCE WORK
DAY 7		REST

It's just business but take it personally.

WEEK 30 - DAY 1

Date:

Focus: Strength

SLEEP   Total Time _____

Quality   1   2   3   4   5

MOBILITY

STRENGTH   90% 1RM   4 Sets   8-10 Reps

Squat   Wt ___ / Reps ___   Wt ___ / Reps ___   Wt ___ / Reps ___   Wt ___ / Reps ___

Deadlift   Wt ___ / Reps ___   Wt ___ / Reps ___   Wt ___ / Reps ___   Wt ___ / Reps ___

OHP   Wt ___ / Reps ___   Wt ___ / Reps ___   Wt ___ / Reps ___   Wt ___ / Reps ___

2-4 minutes rest between sets

NUTRITION   GOAL

TOTAL CALORIES: _____   _____

GRAMS OF PROTEIN: _____   _____

HYDRATION: _____   _____

READING: _____

RESEARCH: _____

WEEK 30 – DAY 2
Date:
Focus: Endurance

SLEEP   Total Time   _____
          Quality   1   2   3   4   5

MOBILITY

ENDURANCE – 5x5   5 mile ruck   55 pounds
            Time: _____
             100 Squats   with ruck
      Run   5 mile run
            Time: _____
             100 Squats   without ruck

Cognition Prompt: See to remember. Pay particular attention to the route and direction you travel. What are the twists, turns, and bends in the path that you took or chose not to take? When you complete you exercise for the day, take a notebook page and see how detailed you can re-create this path and some of the things that occurred to you at key landmarks.

Socks: _____   Boots: _____
Hotspots: _____

NUTRITION   GOAL
      TOTAL CALORIES: _____ ____
    GRAMS OF PROTEIN: _____ ____
        HYDRATION: _____ ____

READING: _____

RESEARCH: _____

WEEK 30 - DAY 3
Date:
Focus: Strength & Recovery

SLEEP   Total Time   _____

               Quality   1   2   3   4   5

MOBILITY

STRENGTH   90% 1RM   4 Sets   8-10 Reps

	Wt	/	Reps	Wt	/	Reps	Wt	/	Reps	Wt	/	Reps
Bench												
Row												
Shrug												

2-4 minutes rest between sets

ENDURANCE   35 min run   Zone 1

              Mileage: _____   Recovery

              Avg HR: _____

NUTRITION   GOAL

           TOTAL CALORIES: _____ _____

      GRAMS OF PROTEIN: _____ _____

               HYDRATION: _____ _____

READING: _____

RESEARCH: _____

WEEK 30 - DAY 4
Date:
Focus: Endurance

SLEEP   Total Time   _____

           Quality   1   2   3   4   5

MOBILITY

ENDURANCE - 5x5   5 mile ruck   55 pounds

             Time: _____

                      100 Squats   with ruck

        Run   5 mile run

             Time: _____

                      100 Squats   without ruck

Cognition Prompt: Explore any pain, unpleasantness, or discomfort you experience during this training day.
What does this pain, and your willingness to experience it, tell you about what matters to you? How can this pain help you grow or develop? How can you learn from this pain?

Socks: _____   Boots: _____

Hotspots: _____

NUTRITION   GOAL

            TOTAL CALORIES: _____ _____

        GRAMS OF PROTEIN: _____ _____

                HYDRATION: _____ _____

READING: _____

RESEARCH: _____

WEEK 30 - DAY 5
Date:
Focus: Strength

SLEEP   Total Time _____
            Quality   1   2   3   4   5

MOBILITY

STRENGTH   90% 1RM   4 Sets   8-10 Reps

Squat Wt / Reps   Wt / Reps   Wt / Reps   Wt / Reps

Deadlift Wt / Reps   Wt / Reps   Wt / Reps   Wt / Reps

OHP Wt / Reps   Wt / Reps   Wt / Reps   Wt / Reps

2-4 minutes rest between sets

NUTRITION   GOAL
            TOTAL CALORIES: _____   _____
            GRAMS OF PROTEIN: _____   _____
            HYDRATION: _____   _____

READING: _____

RESEARCH: _____

WEEK 30 – DAY 6
Date:
Focus: Endurance

SLEEP   Total Time   _____
            Quality   1   2   3   4   5

MOBILITY

ENDURANCE - 5x5   5 mile ruck   55 pounds
                    Time: _____
                             100 Squats   with ruck
            Run   5 mile run
                    Time: _____
                             100 Squats   without ruck

Cognition Prompt: Feel the temperature of your environment. Are you: hot, warm, comfortable, cool, cold, etc.? What sensations make you more aware of the temperature and how it affects you? Do you notice the temperature of the air as you breathe in/out? Is there a breeze or fan blowing on your skin? Is your choice of clothing appropriate for maintain your current level of comfort?

Socks: _____   Boots: _____
Hotspots: _____

NUTRITION   GOAL
        TOTAL CALORIES: _____ _____
      GRAMS OF PROTEIN: _____ _____
             HYDRATION: _____ _____

READING: _____

RESEARCH: _____

WEEK 30 – DAY 7
Date:
Focus: Rest

SLEEP   Total Time   _____

             Quality   1   2   3   4   5

MOBILITY

SUMMARY	SLEEP	CALORIES	PROTEIN	HYDRATION
Day 1				
Day 2				
Day 3				
Day 4				
Day 5				
Day 6				
Day 7				

NUTRITION   GOAL

            TOTAL CALORIES: _____ ___

         GRAMS OF PROTEIN: _____ ___

                 HYDRATION: _____ ___

NEXT WEEK TRAINING FOCUS: _____

_____

_____

WEEK 31 - SUMMARY

Your last speed work session, a recovery run, and two 5x5s. Your final skill
session. Make it count.

DAY 1	MOBILITY 1	STRENGTH WORK
DAY 2	MOBILITY 2	ENDURANCE WORK
DAY 3	MOBILITY 1	STRENGTH & RECOVERY
DAY 4	MOBILITY 2	ENDURANCE WORK
DAY 5	MOBILITY 1	STRENGTH & SPEED
DAY 6	MOBILITY 2	SKILLS WORK
DAY 7		REST

How could you live and have no story to tell?

Date:

Focus: Strength

SLEEP   Total Time   _____

               Quality   1   2   3   4   5

MOBILITY

STRENGTH   90% 1RM   4 Sets   8-10 Reps

	Wt / Reps	Wt / Reps	Wt / Reps	Wt / Reps
Bench				
Row				
Shrug				

2-4 minutes rest between sets

EMERGING LIMITATIONS: _____

EMERGING CAPABILITIES: _____

NUTRITION   GOAL

        TOTAL CALORIES: _____ ____

    GRAMS OF PROTEIN: _____ ____

            HYDRATION: _____ ____

READING: _____

RESEARCH: _____

WEEK 31 - DAY 2
Date:
Focus: Endurance

SLEEP   Total Time   _____

            Quality   1   2   3   4   5

MOBILITY

ENDURANCE - 5x5   5 mile ruck   55 pounds

            Time: _____

                 100 Squats   with ruck

       Run   5 mile run

            Time: _____

                 100 Squats   without ruck

Cognition Prompt: Study any other people who you encounter today during your workout. As you pass them or see them, make a point to focus on their facial features (clothing, height, eight, etc.). What are the things that stand out to you? What inferences might you make about this person? Would you be able to pick them out in a crowd if you saw them again?

Socks: _____   Boots: _____

Hotspots: _____

NUTRITION   GOAL

           TOTAL CALORIES: _____ _____

        GRAMS OF PROTEIN: _____ _____

                HYDRATION: _____ _____

READING: _____

RESEARCH: _____

WEEK 31 - DAY 3
Date:
Focus: Strength and Endurance

SLEEP   Total Time   _____
           Quality   1   2   3   4   5

MOBILITY

STRENGTH   90% 1RM   4 Sets   8-10 Reps

	Wt	/	Reps	Wt	/	Reps	Wt	/	Reps	Wt	/	Reps
Squat												
Deadlift												
OHP												

2-4 minutes rest between sets

ENDURANCE   35 min run   Zone 1
           Mileage: _____   Recovery
           Avg HR: _____

NUTRITION   GOAL
        TOTAL CALORIES: _____ _____
    GRAMS OF PROTEIN: _____ _____
           HYDRATION: _____ _____

READING: _____

RESEARCH: _____

SLEEP   Total Time   _____

              Quality   1   2   3   4   5

MOBILITY

ENDURANCE - 5x5   5 mile ruck   55 pounds

              Time: _____

                   100 Squats   with ruck

       Run   5 mile run

              Time: _____

                   100 Squats   without ruck

Cognition Prompt: Reflect on the Nasty Nick (or similar type obstacle course).
What are the most common areas your attention gets directed to?
Which things are relevant and relate to your effective execution of this task, and which things
are merely 'noise' or distractors?

Socks: _____   Boots: _____

Hotspots: _____

NUTRITION   GOAL

        TOTAL CALORIES: _____ _____

      GRAMS OF PROTEIN: _____ _____

             HYDRATION: _____ _____

READING: _____

RESEARCH: _____

Date:
Focus: Strength & Speed

SLEEP   Total Time   _____
                    Quality   1   2   3   4   5

MOBILITY

STRENGTH   90% 1RM   4 Sets   8-10 Reps

	Wt	/	Reps	Wt	/	Reps	Wt	/	Reps	Wt	/	Reps
Bench												
Row												
Shrug												

2-4 minutes rest between sets

SPEED   Run   8 x 400 - Z4
                                            1:2 work:rest

NUTRITION   GOAL
              TOTAL CALORIES: _____ _____
       GRAMS OF PROTEIN: _____ _____
                  HYDRATION: _____ _____

READING: _____

RESEARCH: _____

SLEEP   Total Time   _____

            Quality   1   2   3   4   5

MOBILITY

SKILLS   From Menu

NUTRITION   GOAL

        TOTAL CALORIES: _____ _____

    GRAMS OF PROTEIN: _____ _____

            HYDRATION: _____ _____

READING: _____

RESEARCH: _____

WEEK 31 – DAY 7

Date:

Focus: Rest

SLEEP   Total Time   _____

Quality   1   2   3   4   5

MOBILITY

SUMMARY	SLEEP	CALORIES	PROTEIN	HYDRATION
Day 1				
Day 2				
Day 3				
Day 4				
Day 5				
Day 6				
Day 7				

NUTRITION   GOAL

TOTAL CALORIES: _____ _____

GRAMS OF PROTEIN: _____ _____

HYDRATION: _____ _____

NEXT WEEK TRAINING FOCUS: _____

WEEK 32 - SUMMARY

It is not because things are difficult that we do not dare; it is because we do not dare that things are difficult. – Seneca

DAY 1	MOBILITY 1	STRENGTH WORK
DAY 2	MOBILITY 2	ENDURANCE WORK
DAY 3	MOBILITY 1	STRENGTH & RECOVERY
DAY 4	MOBILITY 2	ENDURANCE WORK
DAY 5	MOBILITY 1	STRENGTH WORK
DAY 6	MOBILITY 2	ENDURANCE WORK
DAY 7		REST

100% or nothing.

WEEK 32 - DAY 1

Date:

Focus: Strength

SLEEP   Total Time _____

              Quality   1   2   3   4   5

MOBILITY

STRENGTH   90% 1RM   4 Sets   8-10 Reps

Squat   Wt / Reps   Wt / Reps   Wt / Reps   Wt / Reps

Deadlift Wt / Reps   Wt / Reps   Wt / Reps   Wt / Reps

OHP   Wt / Reps   Wt / Reps   Wt / Reps   Wt / Reps

2-4 minutes rest between sets

NUTRITION   GOAL

TOTAL CALORIES: _____ _____

GRAMS OF PROTEIN: _____ _____

HYDRATION: _____ _____

READING: _____

RESEARCH: _____

SLEEP   Total Time   _____

              Quality   1   2   3   4   5

MOBILITY

ENDURANCE - 5x5   5 mile ruck   55 pounds
                  Time: _____
                          100 Squats   with ruck
          Run   5 mile run
                  Time: _____
                          100 Squats   without ruck

Cognition Prompt: Reflect on the task of Land Navigation.
What are the most common areas your attention gets directed to?
Which things are relevant and relate to your effective execution of this task, and which things
are merely 'noise' or distractors?

Socks: _____   Boots: _____
Hotspots: _____

NUTRITION   GOAL
              TOTAL CALORIES: _____ _____
          GRAMS OF PROTEIN: _____ _____
                  HYDRATION: _____ _____

READING: _____

RESEARCH: _____

WEEK 32 - DAY 3
Date:
Focus: Strength

SLEEP   Total Time   _____
             Quality   1   2   3   4   5

MOBILITY

STRENGTH   90% 1RM   4 Sets   8-10 Reps

Bench Wt / Reps   Wt / Reps   Wt / Reps   Wt / Reps
_____

Row   Wt / Reps   Wt / Reps   Wt / Reps   Wt / Reps
_____

Shrug Wt / Reps   Wt / Reps   Wt Reps   Wt / Reps
_____

2-4 minutes rest between sets

ENDURANCE   35 min run   Zone 1
               Mileage: _____   Recovery
               Avg HR: _____

NUTRITION   GOAL
        TOTAL CALORIES: _____ _____
      GRAMS OF PROTEIN: _____ _____
             HYDRATION: _____ _____

READING: _____

RESEARCH: _____

WEEK 32 – DAY 4
Date:
Focus: Endurance

SLEEP   Total Time   _____

Quality   1   2   3   4   5

MOBILITY

ENDURANCE - 5x5   5 mile ruck   55 pounds

Time: _____

100 Squats   with ruck

Run   5 mile run

Time: _____

100 Squats   without ruck

Cognition Prompt: Reflect on team week.
You will need to work collaboratively with other candidates, some of which you will not agree with or get along with.
What are your triggers that typically interfere with your capacity to work well with others?
What are the cues that allow you to ID them before they get in the way?

Socks: _____   Boots: _____

Hotspots: _____

NUTRITION   GOAL

TOTAL CALORIES: _____ _____

GRAMS OF PROTEIN: _____ _____

HYDRATION: _____ _____

READING: _____

RESEARCH: _____

WEEK 32 - DAY 5
Date:
Focus: Strength

SLEEP   Total Time   _____

              Quality   1   2   3   4   5

MOBILITY

STRENGTH   90% 1RM   4 Sets   8-10 Reps

Squat	Wt	/	Reps	Wt	/	Reps	Wt	/	Reps	Wt	/	Reps

Deadlift	Wt	/	Reps	Wt	/	Reps	Wt	/	Reps	Wt	/	Reps

OHP	Wt	/	Reps	Wt	/	Reps	Wt	/	Reps	Wt	/	Reps

2-4 minutes rest between sets

NUTRITION   GOAL

              TOTAL CALORIES: _____ _____

       GRAMS OF PROTEIN: _____ _____

                  HYDRATION: _____ _____

READING: _____

RESEARCH: _____

WEEK 32 – DAY 6
Date:
Focus: Endurance

SLEEP   Total Time   _____

               Quality   1   2   3   4   5

MOBILITY

ENDURANCE – 5x5   5 mile ruck   55 pounds

              Time: _____

                      100 Squats   with ruck

        Run   5 mile run

              Time: _____

                      100 Squats   without ruck

Cognition Prompt: We did this one already. Has your answer changed?   **Why are you going to SFAS?**
If you had to boil it down to 1 or 2 specific reasons, what would they be?

Socks: _____   Boots: _____

Hotspots: _____

NUTRITION   GOAL

         TOTAL CALORIES: _____ _____

     GRAMS OF PROTEIN: _____ _____

             HYDRATION: _____ _____

READING: _____

RESEARCH: _____

WEEK 32 – DAY 7

Date:

Focus: Rest

SLEEP   Total Time   _____

              Quality   1   2   3   4   5

MOBILITY

SUMMARY	SLEEP	CALORIES	PROTEIN	HYDRATION
Day 1				
Day 2				
Day 3				
Day 4				
Day 5				
Day 6				
Day 7				

NUTRITION   GOAL

TOTAL CALORIES: _____ _____

GRAMS OF PROTEIN: _____ _____

HYDRATION: _____ _____

You're ready. Go to war.

SKILLS MENU

Knot Tying – rope, tubular nylon
Rope Climbing
Mantling
Balance – loaded, unloaded, asymmetrically loaded, at height
Handstands
Comfort with heights
Comfort with enclosed spaces
Underhand Ball Catch – small, large, weighted
Underhand Ball Throw – small, large, weighted
Overhand Throw – small, large, weighted
Overhand Catch – small, large, weighted
Juggling - hand-eye coordination
Explosive Jumping – loaded, unloaded
Dynamic Landing – loaded, unloaded
Falling – forward, backwards, side
Bike Riding
Swimming
Tree Climbing
Turkish Get Up
Pistol Squats
Footwork – Agility Ladder - forward , backwards , lateral
Hopping - forward , backwards , lateral
Turning - loaded, unloaded
Sprawling - loaded, unloaded
Jumping rope -forward , backwards , lateral
Dribbling - forward , backwards , lateral
Cone Weave - forward , backwards , lateral
Hurdles, mini hurdles - forward , backwards , lateral
Shuffle runs - forward , backwards , lateral
Pit Stop – How fast can you change socks on a ruck workout

MAX HEART RATE						
220 minus Age						
	50%	60%	70%	80%	85%	90%
150	75	90	105	120	127.5	135
155	77.5	93	108.5	124	132	140
160	80	96	112	128	136	144
165	82.5	99	115.5	132	140	149
170	85	102	119	136	144.5	153
175	87.5	105	122.5	140	149	157.5
180	90	108	126	144	153	162
185	92.5	111	129.5	148	157	166.5
190	95	114	133	152	161.5	171
195	97.5	117	136.5	156	166	175.5
200	100	120	140	160	170	180

PACE (hh:mm:ss)			
1/4 Mile (Lap)	Mile	5 Mile	12 Mile
:01:00	:04:00	:20:00	:48:00
:01:15	:05:00	:25:00	:60:00
:01:30	:06:00	:30:00	1:12:00
:01:45	:07:00	:35:00	1:24:00
:02:00	:08:00	:40:00	1:36:00
:02:15	:09:00	:45:00	1:48:00
:02:30	:10:00	:50:00	2:00:00
:02:45	:11:00	:55:00	2:12:00
:03:00	:12:00	1:00:00	2:24:00
:03:15	:13:00	1:05:00	2:36:00
:03:30	:14:00	1:10:00	2:48:00
:03:45	:15:00	1:15:00	3:00:00
:04:00	:16:00	1:20:00	3:12:00
:04:15	:17:00	1:25:00	3:24:00
:04:30	:18:00	1:30:00	3:36:00
:04:45	:19:00	1:35:00	3:48:00
:05:00	:20:00	1:40:00	4:00:00

Lifting Percentage

Weight (1RM)	75.00%	80.00%	85.00%	90.00%	95.00%	Weight (1RM)	75.00%	80.00%	85.00%	90.00%	95.00%
75	56	60	64	68	71	185	139	148	157	167	176
80	60	64	68	72	76	190	143	152	162	171	181
85	64	68	72	77	81	195	146	156	166	176	185
90	68	72	77	81	86	200	150	160	170	180	190
95	71	76	81	86	90	205	154	164	174	185	195
100	75	80	85	90	95	210	158	168	179	189	200
105	79	84	89	95	100	215	161	172	183	194	204
110	83	88	94	99	105	220	165	176	187	198	209
115	86	92	98	104	109	225	169	180	191	203	214
120	90	96	102	108	114	230	173	184	196	207	219
125	94	100	106	113	119	235	176	188	200	212	223
130	98	104	111	117	124	240	180	192	204	216	228
135	101	108	115	122	128	245	184	196	208	221	233
140	105	112	119	126	133	250	188	200	213	225	238
145	109	116	123	131	138	255	191	204	217	230	242
150	113	120	128	135	143	260	195	208	221	234	247
155	116	124	132	140	147	265	199	212	225	239	252
160	120	128	136	144	152	270	203	216	230	243	257
165	124	132	140	149	157	275	206	220	234	248	261
170	128	136	145	153	162	280	210	224	238	252	266
175	131	140	149	158	166	285	214	228	242	257	271
180	135	144	153	162	171	290	218	232	247	261	276

Lifting Percentage

Weight (1RM)	75.00%	80.00%	85.00%	90.00%	95.00%	Weight (1RM)	75.00%	80.00%	85.00%	90.00%	95.00%
295	221	236	251	266	280	405	304	324	344	365	385
300	225	240	255	270	285	410	308	328	349	369	390
305	229	244	259	275	290	415	311	332	353	374	394
310	233	248	264	279	295	420	315	336	357	378	399
315	236	252	268	284	299	425	319	340	361	383	404
320	240	256	272	288	304	430	323	344	366	387	409
325	244	260	276	293	309	435	326	348	370	392	413
330	248	264	281	297	314	440	330	352	374	396	418
335	251	268	285	302	318	445	334	356	378	401	423
340	255	272	289	306	323	450	338	360	383	405	428
345	259	276	293	311	328	455	341	364	387	410	432
350	263	280	298	315	333	460	345	368	391	414	437
355	266	284	302	320	337	465	349	372	395	419	442
360	270	288	306	324	342	470	353	376	400	423	447
365	274	292	310	329	347	475	356	380	404	428	451
370	278	296	315	333	352	480	360	384	408	432	456
375	281	300	319	338	356	485	364	388	412	437	461
380	285	304	323	342	361	490	368	392	417	441	466
385	289	308	327	347	366	495	371	396	421	446	470
390	293	312	332	351	371	500	375	400	425	450	475
395	296	316	336	356	375	505	379	404	429	455	480
400	300	320	340	360	380	510	383	408	434	459	485

Functional Movement Screening

0: You feel any pain at all
1: You can do the move, but not very well
2. You can do the move, but you need to compensate in some way.
3. You can perfectly master the move.

DEEP SQUAT   0   1   2   3

- Hold a dowel rod above your head. Then, squat as low as possible while keeping good form (head looking forward, chest upright, knees pointing forward).
- The goal is for your upper torso to be parallel with your shins and knees and dowel aligned over your feet.

INLINE LUNGE   0   1   2   3

- Hold the dowel behind your back with one hand near your neck and the other toward your lower back. Then, with your feet about hip-width apart and facing forward, step one foot back and lower it until it hits the floor. Use a balance pad for extra support if you need it.
- You're looking for the dowel to stay in place. Your torso to remain still, and your feet to face forward as your back knee lowers.

HURDLE STEP   0   1   2   3

- Hold the dowel across your shoulders in front of a hurdle. Now, step over the hurdle with one leg, touching the heel to the floor. Return to starting position. Then, repeat on the other side.
- You're looking for balance and for your upper body to remain neutral as you move your legs.

SHOULDER MOBILITY   0   1   2   3

- Reach your hands behind your back simultaneously, putting one over your shoulder and the other around your back reaching up. Repeat on the other side.
- Your goal is to get your hands as close together as possible.

ACTIVE STRAIGHT LEG RAISE   0   1   2   3

- Lie on your back with your arms at your sides. Raise one leg as high as you can while keeping your knee straight. The other leg remains on the floor.
- You're looking at how high you can raise your leg while keeping your other leg on the floor.

TRUNK STABILITY PUSH UP   0   1   2   3

- Get in a plank position and perform a push-up, going as far to the ground as possible before pushing yourself back into starting position. Cushion your hands using a yoga foam wedge block.
- Your goal is to get your chest to the ground and back up while keeping your body in a straight line.

ROTATIONAL STABILITY   0   1   2   3

- Put your knees down, so you are on all fours. Simultaneously raise your right leg and arm until they are parallel to the floor. Next, touch your right elbow to your right knee. Extend your arm and leg again, then put them on the floor before repeating on the left side.
- Your goal is to keep your elbow aligned with your knee and to do the move without twisting your torso. Pay attention to the differences between your left and right sides.

Made in the USA
Las Vegas, NV
28 May 2024

90463381R00252